ABOUT THE AUTHORS

Simon Cook was born in India in 1938 and was educated in England. He joined the Royal Marines in 1957, serving with the Commandos until he specialised in physical fitness in 1963, being trained at the Royal Naval and Royal Marines physical training schools. When he wrote this book he was commanding the Royal Marines Physical Training School at Deal in Kent and was responsible for training Commando physical fitness instructors and for research on methods of getting and keeping fit. After further service, including a year in command of the Military Garrison in the Falkland Islands, he joined Local Government as a Recreation and Leisure Officer. He is a hockey international and a Fellow of the British Association of Physical Training. He is currently working for the Sedgemoor District Council in Somerset.

Tony Toms was born in Durham in 1941. He joined the Royal Marines in 1961 and served with the Commandos all over the world, including active service during the Aden emergency. He specialised in physical fitness and was the youngest Staff Instructor ever appointed at the Royal Marines Physical Training School. He joined Hartlepool Football Club as coach and trainer in 1972 and immediately established his team as one of the fittest in the league. In 1975, he moved to Gillingham Football Club and his methods were so successful that Kent County Cricket Club engaged him as their trainer, a position he still holds during the summer season. He moved to Sheffield Wednesday in early 1976 when this famous club appeared doomed to relegation to the fourth division, and hit the headlines with his dedicated approach to physical fitness. Against all the odds, the club avoided relegation and he remains their trainer and Assistant Manager today. He played rugby for Richmond and the South of England and has representative honours in several sports. He runs an enormously successful physical fitness class and is, himself, supremely fit.

Royal Marine Commando 7 Exercises

SIMON COOK and TONY TOMS

With Forewords by Alan Knott and Bob Stokoe

SPHERE BOOKS LIMITED
30/32 Gray's Inn Road, London WC1X 8JL

First published in Great Britain by Sphere Books Ltd 1973
Copyright © Simon Cook and Tony Toms 1973
Reprinted 1977, 1978 (twice), 1979

TRADE
MARK

Set in Monotype Baskerville

Printed in Great Britain by
Hazell Watson & Vine Ltd
Aylesbury, Bucks

FOREWORD

Being physically fit is one of the requirements of a top class sportsman and I have always been very interested in the subject. I am, therefore, delighted to be able to recommend this book to anyone who wishes to get and keep fit.

This book contains a simple programme for getting fit, for maintaining fitness at a satisfactory level (page 96) and a way to achieve what the authors describe as 'super fitness'!

The book is, in fact, aimed at putting physical fitness within the grasp of virtually anybody who recognises the authors' contention that being physically fit can help you to lead a healthier and happier life.

I can vouch for the excellence of Tony Toms' practical work on fitness from personal experience of his training the Kent County Cricket Team.

A. P. E. Knott
(Kent and England)

This book by two Royal Marine Physical Training Instructors is about a subject rarely attempted on so broad a basis. Publications in this field are usually written for those specialists who wish to be supremely fit for one particular sport.

Authors Captain Simon Cook, a P.T. Officer, and Tony Toms, an ex-P.T. Staff Instructor who now trains footballers for Sheffield Wednesday Football Club, have drawn deeply upon their knowledge of the human body and its capabilities.

From this informative book the average man can learn to keep himself fitter and achieve something worthwhile—a healthy body.

Today's starchy foods and polluted atmospheres take their toll on a man's body. For the man in the street health farms, specialist health foods and suchlike gimmicks are beyond his time and his purse. It is very much a 'do-it-yourself' business for him but he must be given the 'know-how'.

So far there has been no simple guide to the problem of keeping fit. Now there is, with this book which I have much pleasure in recommending to anyone interested in making better use of something which we all take for granted—our bodies.

To conclude—the authors, as well as being outstanding performers in several sports, have ample qualifications to have written this book. They have a huge background experience of training men to do many physical tasks and fortunately they have been able to express this experience in layman's terms for the benefit of all.

Bob Stokoe

ACKNOWLEDGEMENTS

When we know that we have enjoyed the help and co-operation of so many people, it is difficult to be exact and yet brief in giving our acknowledgements. To the Royal Marines and Royal Navy for both training us and permitting us to publish, go our first thanks. Next we are pleased to record our appreciation to Tyne Tees Television, and particularly to Mr. Roderick Griffiths, who prompted the original idea of television exercises, for their co-operation in releasing the copyright. We thank the *Sunday Times* and particularly Mr. Allan Hall for publicising the complete Commando 7 Series and for subsequently releasing their half of the copyright on the Look "Keep Fit Commando Style" Wall Chart and the two fitness maintenance tables. Many individuals freely gave of their time and first we acknowledge the original vetting of the *Commando 7 Exercises* script prior to the screening on television by Surgeon Commander D. E. McKay, MD, CHb, DPH(p). The chore of proof-reading the book was willingly undertaken by fellow physical trainer, Mr. Ken Wilson and a remedial gymnast, Sgt. C. F. L. Bell, and we gratefully acknowledge their work. The diagrams were mainly created by Mr. Rodney Kilbeè with help from Sgt. H. R. E. Lee. For the enormous task of re-typing numerous drafts and then for completely re-typing the final script copy, we both acknowledge with gratitude the work of Mrs. Erica Cook. We hope that we have not inadvertently omitted the names of any persons who gave us advice or help, but we hope that we have expressed our thanks to those who were most involved in creating this book. Finally we appreciate permission to quote from C. H. McCloy's *Fitness for What* in Physical Education; and Dr. M. F. Graham's *Prescription for Life* (published in New York by the David McKay Company).

CONTENTS

INTRODUCTION

Modern society has created enormous health problems, many of which are directly related to poor standards of physical fitness. While great advances have been made on almost every sociological and scientific front and although living standards in the Western world keep rising, the human body is being allowed to suffer from neglect. This book is about that neglect.

We aim to explain why a human body needs to be treated with care. We want you to know how your body works and why it needs the benefit of regular and *vigorous* exercise. A human body that is not exercised regularly becomes inefficient and eventually breaks down through ill health or premature old age. The picture is all too simple and very clear.

We are, essentially, practical trainers rather than theorists. We do not pretend to have the detailed and lengthy training given to scientists, doctors and physiologists. We are only expert in the specific field of training and teaching people to be physically fit.

Both of us were trained within the service of the Royal Naval and Royal Marines Physical Training Branches to actively train men to be fit enough to join the Royal Marines Commandos. After training we both enjoyed the benefit of several years' hard practical work training boys and men straight from civilian life in fitness and sport.

The Commando 7 Exercise routines were originally written by us when working on the staff of the Royal Marines Physical Training School, for a small independent television company (Tyne Tees) who were producing a pilot programme on practical fitness for the general public in the North East. The exercises were an immediate success and the *Sunday Times* published the full series of routines over ten weeks in 1972.

The volume of correspondence which emanated from the public as a result of both the provincial television showing and the national publication confirmed that there was a great interest in a fitness programme which could be attempted by virtually anybody. It was for this reason that we decided to prepare a book on fitness based on the now proven Commando 7 Exercises, which could become a guide for everybody. This book is the result.

In the early chapters you will learn about your most valuable possession, your body, and about what it is capable of doing provided that it is trained properly. We explain why the Commando 7 Exercises were written in the way they have been and how anybody, however unfit, can do them. We illustrate how one feels so much better and is much healthier if the body is physically fit and after giving the entire Commando 7 routines for both men and women, we present ideas on maintaining fitness which are both enjoyable and effective.

No book on fitness would be complete without some comments on nutrition, because both eating and drinking habits help towards the general destructive attitude of many people to their own physical shape and state. The relevant information is included where necessary, although we would argue that the fitter the subject the more capable he or she will be of indulging in that favourite, but potentially damaging, food or drink.

The penultimate chapter of the book is aimed at showing some of the heights to which the body can climb. The contents of this chapter are included for general interest and to provide a challenge which those who are young enough may aspire to meet.

The aim of the pages that follow is simple but important. We give you the reasons why it is so very necessary to be physically fit, we provide you with the methods by which you can reach and keep to the healthy state. We believe that physical fitness is vital to the enjoyment and fulfilment of life itself. We offer a key with which to open the door to this better life.

CHAPTER I

YOUR MOST VALUABLE POSSESSION—YOUR BODY

The body with which the human being starts his life is an efficient machine. It is perfectly designed for life, except when some mischance of nature or science affects the initial production process. For the great majority, however, this body is their most valuable possession. It is the basis of life. Unfortunately, the very progress which is proclaimed as the years go by has brought in its wake a widespread abuse of the body machinery. The result is that the most advanced industrial countries are peopled by humans with inefficient bodies that are receptive to both sickness and injury.

Before considering the twentieth-century human body, it is worth looking back at history and considering one of the evolutionary processes which influenced the development of modern man. This first big breakthrough in physical development came when our gorilla-like ancestors discovered the ability to walk on two legs instead of on four. This evolution gave man the facility of being able to use his hands and therefore handle tools, make and move objects and defend himself in a different manner than hitherto. This early example of body evolution led to the human arm being developed and shows us how the regular use of a muscle or group of muscles encourages the health and growth of those muscles. One only has to compare the arms of a manual worker with those of a man whose job needs only a limited amount of arm work to confirm the accuracy of this assertion.

Gradually the body of modern man evolved. It was required to carry out certain activities and functions in order to live and survive in the various periods of history. As the environmental conditions of life changed so did the human body, by degrees, adapt its capacity and method of physical work, with the emphasis changing and with specific muscles and joints altering their characteristics. This change in physical evolution is confirmed by a comparison between the average human living in modern Western society and his equivalent from an underdeveloped part of the world.

With this brief glimpse into the past it becomes easier to look at the average human body living in the sophisticated civilisation of today. It has developed in accordance with the needs of the society in which it lives; it is thus that the modern human body machine has evolved to meet the stresses and strains of today.

The human animal is made up of bone, muscle, fat and blood. Something like 70% of the average male is, in fact, water. There are two hundred and six bones and six hundred and thirty-nine muscles in this mixture and about 40% of the actual body weight is made up of muscle.

Working this complex system is a complicated brain, which works through the central nervous system and drives the whole affair. This, then, without attempting to analyse the cells and tissue make-up which form these component parts, is the body which you use to live on earth.

The tissues of the body are arranged to form organs and these are grouped into systems. It is these systems which give you the actual working body. The systems control the thought and response process, metabolism and growth, respiration, nutrition, excretion, the movement of materials such as food around the body, reproduction and all external locomotion.

During the course of our lives our bodies are replenished by the replacement of worn-out tissues. Proteins, specifically body proteins, are replaced every twenty-eight days. Blood make-up is changed regularly. Muscle tissue is broken down and repaired daily. We can therefore see from all this activity that the body renews itself entirely every few months.

Some of these tissues (cells) have the quality of being able to repair themselves extremely quickly. The muscle tissues for instance can repair themselves in this way. Consequently, muscle can be manoeuvred through exercise to develop or shape up very quickly. The brain cells, on the other hand, renew slowly and when damaged show very little regeneration. It is because of this rapid response of the muscles that there is no better way of helping the body than by regular exercise.

Almost all the necessary functioning systems of the body are controlled by muscles, the greatest of which is the heart. This organ is in reality a double pump which operate separately from each other. Its function is to pump oxygen-loaded blood around the body and to the areas where energy is required. The blood goes on its journey and gradually loses or delivers the oxygen, before returning via the heart for replenishment with more oxygen from the lungs. The renewed blood returns to the heart before being dispatched back on its energy-giving journey around the body. The whole cycle takes about 0·8 seconds when the heart beat is around a norm 72–75 beats a minute. The efficient working of the heart and the lungs is the basis of all physical fitness training.

When the body is completely at rest the heart is at its resting rate (basic metabolic rate) which means that just enough energy is being demanded through muscular action in order to breathe. When the body is involved in vigorous exercise, then the heart rate rises and pumps energy, in the form of oxygen-carrying blood, to that part of the body that demands it in order that it can work. The greater the demand, the more the heart and lungs work. In the physically fit person the capacity of the heart and lungs to work is much greater than in the unfit and the recovery from the stresses of that work will be much swifter. The message is clear. The heart and lungs cannot be allowed to deteriorate through lack of work or they will not be able to work safely when called upon unexpectedly.

It is interesting to note that the emotions can by themselves work the heart alone and it is reckoned that the pulse rate of a person making a speech can be around 180 beats a minute! Unfortunately for many a businessman this method of raising the pulse will not provide much value to the body from a physiological angle, because the muscles are not being worked and therefore the whole body system is not involved. An analogy is the motor car that has its engine raced while stationary.

Having now established that the body is a complicated machine, the engine room of which is the heart, it is important to remind ourselves that society gives modern man every chance to abuse this

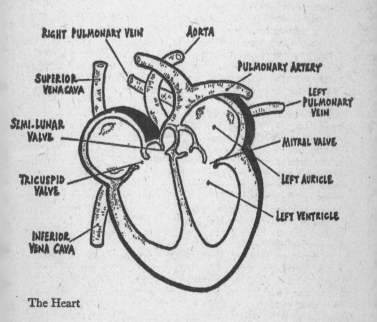

The Heart

body. One of the main ways in which this is done is, quite apart from a disregard of physical exercise, by self-pollution. By this one means over-eating, bad eating habits, smoking, drinking and even giving the body insufficient rest. For those unlucky enough to live in a heavy industrial area, the very act of breathing is a form of this self pollution. All these are problems of the modern environment and they add to the pressure on the human frame which is frequently not physically efficient enough to cope. The result is a failure to combat these extra pressures and the body becomes receptive to sickness, injury and even to mental collapse. It is appreciated that industrialisation and the urbanisation that is increasingly taking place is reducing the demands for the human to take exercise in order to live. It is also recognised that the advent of motorised transport and the push-button era has aggravated the problem and meant that many people barely need to use any physical energy to live. What must now be realised is that the reduction of this physical work load is actively harmful to the human race. Doctors are increasingly becoming aware that this lack of physical capacity is lowering resistance to acute and chronic diseases and probably affects longevity and is certainly bad for the general physical well being of the human race. It is a dangerous situation.

The biggest single killer illness in the western world is heart disease. It is reckoned that by next year one million Americans will have died of it and that in the United Kingdom the figure will be over 200,000. One of the main reasons for coronary heart disease is the build up of fatty substances (cholesterol) in the access to and on the valves within the heart. A blockage forms and the arteries harden, thus reducing the size of the access to the heart and thereby setting up a back pressure of blood. Eventually the free flow of blood into the heart is stopped and this breaks the cycle of movement necessary to life.

Although it would be unwise to claim that regular exercise could eliminate this plague on our society, because there are too many imponderables involved, doctors are agreed that regular exercise reduces the chances of individuals contracting it. Another of the current bains of the doctor's surgery is the prevalence of back pain and injury, often attributed to the dreaded "slipped disc". The painful inconvenience of back injuries is almost 90% attributable to weak back muscles, a condition which could easily have been avoided by regular exercise. There are of course other examples which could have been taken which would illustrate the connection between lack of physical conditioning and some of the most common ailments, but little has yet been proved. One has only to look around and see who in your particular society or circle of acquaintances is susceptible to sickness and injury for the link between physical fitness and health to be abundantly clear.

The importance of your body to you cannot be overstated. If it is

16

maintained in a physically fit and therefore efficient working order then the benefit to you and to your life is incalculable. You will enjoy each day of a long life, with a feeling of well being, with a happy confidence that you are right in treating your body as your most valuable possession.

CHAPTER II

A BACKCLOTH TO YOUR PHYSICAL TRAINING PLAN

Before launching the body into a fitness programme it is useful to consider physical fitness as an aim and as an end. It is a most worthwhile end and one that is desperately important to achieve in order to obtain full value out of living. The training which leads to this goal has a history of gradual development, offers a myriad of methods and suffers from countless definitions. It is therefore necessary to explain this background in order to provide a platform of knowledge on which to build your active and healthy participation in our programme.

From earliest history physical exercise has been used for the education and development of youth. It is certain that ancient China possessed two systems of physical training, one of which served as a training for war and the other which was designed as a method of healing disease and deformity. Evidence exists that the old civilisations of Persia, India, Israel and Japan had methods of physical training, and pictures exist of exercises taking place in ancient Egypt.

Interest in physical exercise reached a peak with the ancient Greeks and in the development of both the mind and the body their civilisation reached the heights. The Olympic Games was, of course, the focal point of their achievements of physical excellence and it is a legacy which their society has bequeathed to the present day. One of the most famous of the events, the pentathlon, provides us with a clue to their theories on physical training. The running and jumping events exercised the legs, the discus and javelin throwing, the arms and shoulders, and wrestling, the torso. They also pioneered a whole series of exercises which are similar to modern gymnastics.

Although the Romans held physical culture as an important part of general education, it never reached a position of any influence in the scheme of their world. The coming of Christianity appeared to kill the waning interest in physical education for a very long time, because the early Christians held the spiritual values as everything, to the exclusion of the physical. Despite this, many great men through the ages emphasised the importance of physical education to the general education of youth. However, little progress was made until the middle of the eighteenth century, when an attempt was made to introduce it in Germany as part of a school curriculum.

A similar system to that used by the Greeks was publicised in 1793 in a book by a German (Gutsmuth—Gymnastics). From this small start a comprehensive system of physical training was gradually developed and linked to the knowledge of the structure and function of the body. The pioneers of this major leap forward were a German named Nachtigall, and his student, a Swede, Pehr Henrie Ling. It was Ling who made a study of anatomy and physiology and perfected what became known as the Swedish System and which was subsequently introduced as a compulsory part of the education syllabus. This system was so good that, with modifications, it was used by the British Services until the 1950s.

This is the broad outline of physical training history. In recent years the interest in the subject has developed at a relatively much faster rate. It would, therefore, be impossible to attempt to discuss the many theories, ideas and attitudes evolved, expressed, experimented with, adopted and published during the past two decades. Most have aimed at either achieving a state of all-round physical fitness or fitness for a specific activity, such as boxing or football. We are only concerned with all-round physical fitness.

Before considering some of the current methods used to obtain the bodily state called physical fitness, we must answer the obvious question: what exactly is physical fitness? The corollary to this is: for what must you be fit? The answer to both these questions has been pontificated upon by students of physical training for years. Probably C. H. McCloy has come the nearest to giving an accurate definition of normal fitness—as a person having sufficient strength and endurance:

"To feel good, to be able to do the work of the day without undue fatigue and reach the end of the day sleepy but not tired, and to be able to meet emergencies adequately."

The emergencies to which he referred are the physical emergencies of everyday life, such as climbing stairs, running for a bus, digging in a garden or lifting an unexpectedly heavy weight. It is these sudden activities that frequently trigger off the coronary or send a patient to the doctor with crippling back pains, simply because the body has been unable to cope with sudden physical effort.

Obviously there is a clear distinction between normal fitness and super or specialised fitness. The very job of work done to live will regulate the amount of exercise you unconsciously take and therefore your standard of physical fitness. We argue that a large percentage of the population are existing in a substandard state of physical working efficiency and are therefore subjecting themselves to an unnecessary health hazard. Too many people do not live within the perimeters of this definition of normal or safe fitness.

In order to achieve a situation where the body is permitted to exist on the right side of the fitness safety barrier, there are several aids available. These are the methods by which the body can become and can keep fit. They should all be used with a reasonable attention to fuel intake (food and drink) and a proper regard for the necessity to rest. These physical conditioning methods are aimed at two things, the cardiovascular and the skeletal muscular systems. Together these systems are involved in the provision of oxygen to the skeletal muscles. Cardiovascular training is therefore the presentation of a challenge to the heart, circulation and the body's respiratory workings. The efficiency with which the oxygen is supplied will regulate body fatigue. Hence we have endurance and stamina. Conversely, the specific working of muscle is aimed primarily at strength in a localised body area, but also relates to the energy delivered, because without oxygen a muscle cannot contract. Both systems are therefore inter-related, although the emphasis may be different in any particular method of physical training.

The four main types of training are aerobics, calisthenics, weight training and circuit training. These each have their own place in any physical training programme. Aerobics is the running, walking and playing games type of exercise. Calisthenics is a free standing exercise programme which is aimed at a general physical conditioning. Weight training is the use of weights to "overload" and provide resistance, thereby developing specific muscular strength and power. The last group is circuit training and this is a series of exercises/activities designed as a circuit around which the subject has to proceed within specific time limits. These limits and the strength of the various stances can be varied according to the individual's requirements and progress.

Any of the types of training employed work on certain principles if they are to be effective. These principles are: overload, progression and regularity. The last two are obvious enough. An exercise programme must be progressive until you have reached your objective and similarly it would be ludicrous to expect success in becoming and keeping fit if you did not exercise regularly.

The overload principle is harder to understand and yet it is important because it forms the basis on which an exercise programme is designed. It means that the body is made to do more physical work that it is used to and is gradually pushed to undertake more work in increasing quantities. As the body manages certain physical work, so the body capacity increases and the overload of work is increased. This is the principle of overload which allied to progression and regularity is behind any successful fitness programme.

The history, developments, methods, and principles of such a vast subject as physical fitness training are difficult to summarise in one chapter, but it is important that we realise the enormity and complexity of the subject. It is only by gaining for ourselves a satisfactory backcloth of knowledge that we can confidently attempt, take and keep to a new pathway to physical fitness.

CHAPTER III

THE WHY, HOW AND WHEN OF THE COMMANDO 7

The pace of life today leaves little time for the average person to exercise the body, however important to his or her well being. It is therefore essential that an exercise programme takes little time and yet is effective, safe and easy to follow.

The various principles of physical fitness were fully considered when the Commando 7 Exercises were being designed and tested at the Royal Marines Physical Training School. The problem of time in a modern society was always evident as being an important factor in persuading people to participate. We must realise this when considering the Commando 7 programme alongside other methods of getting fit.

The comparison is useful because it clarifies the authors' views and gives the reader an opportunity to understand why this plan is proposed and how he can best utilise it to the real benefit of the body.

Any thought that weight training or indeed circuit training is a feasible proposition for a wide public is rejected because of a general lack of suitable facilities and expertise throughout the country. Both methods are generally used for sportsmen, keep-fit enthusiasts and weight watchers, but unless there is a properly qualified physical trainer available to instruct and supervise the application of these methods, then they can be dangerous.

We particularly tend to regard weight training as a specialist form of physical fitness which both needs and requires specialised knowledge for it to be safely used. Opinions vary on its use and while it is certainly true that the development of maximum strength and power is best produced through weight training, it may not be particularly useful in the simple object of obtaining "normal" fitness. One of the authors has practised it both personally and with many subjects, while the other is not a disciple nor does he believe it to be either beneficial or natural to the average human frame. Most people are not aiming at super fitness at this stage and therefore there is no need for weight training.

More relevant to the normal being is the group of exercises which have been termed in recent years as "aerobics". These are running, walking and any sport which employs either activity and works the heart and lungs. The variety of activities which come under this heading are detailed in Chapter VII. This sort of exercise is the finest method of physical conditioning known to man. The problem is that this type of exercise nearly always requires time, space and opportunity. These are commodities which are not always available.

Not only do they suffer from these disadvantages, but they can invite injury to the skeletal muscles and body jointage because the strength and regularity of the activity has been inexpertly selected and planned. It is easy to see how the hard game of football, or the long run after a long lay off, may cause muscles to be pulled and ankles, knees and backs to suffer damage.

The value of the aerobic exercise is unquestioned, but it is the sort of exercise that must be understood. In our plan for the maintenance of general fitness (Chapter VIII) we list and grade activities which are useful and can help you keep fit. That ultimately the aerobic exercise is the best method of fitness training is not doubted, but the body must be prepared and the type of activity well chosen. If you can find the time and the facilities available to walk, run and play games regularly then do so. The more the heart is exercised the better for the body. The words of Dr. M. F. Graham (*Prescription For Life*—published by David McKay Company) are worth recording in this context:

"How can the overeating, harried and hurried, chain smoking white collar worker, bound to his desk, a phone in one hand, a watch in the other, beleaguered with deadlines and trapped in tension, get away from it all: the answer is he can run!"

Because few people can find the time or the space to run, walk or play games regularly, there is clearly a need for something else more convenient as a way to fitness. We believe that the gimmick fitness aid can largely be discounted for general fitness and therefore we must look elsewhere.

The Commando 7 Exercises provide the answer. The progressive exercise routines require little time, no equipment and virtually no space. The aim of the programme is a general physical conditioning of the body and the developing of strength and efficiency of the important muscles and joints of the body.

The Commando 7 Exercises are mainly derived from the exercises which are employed in the early part of the physical training to which recruits to the Royal Marines Commandos are subjected. They are mainly calisthenic and gymnastic and make up a light free standing circuit, which has been suitably modified for the general public. They are designed to be progressive and to introduce a safe degree of overload in them. Although in the initial stages of the programme most subjects will not feel a difficult physical work load, later the challenge and the load increase.

The exercises can literally be carried out anywhere, from your bathroom to your bedroom or wherever you have room to stand or to lie down. Absolutely no equipment is needed and you only have to follow simple instructions, which are clearly illustrated. The routines are safe and virtually anybody over about ten and under about sixty can do the exercises. A detailed medical warning is included in Chapter V and if you are in any doubt about your physical ability to exercise in the Commando 7 way, then you should consult your doctor before starting. However, the experience of many thousands of people who have taken the course indicate that the exercises are set at such a basic level, that provided you keep to the plan of progress then there is no danger.

Any method of physical fitness training must be effective to be of any value. The Commando 7 is remarkably effective. The basic plan is designed to get the subject fit in ten weeks. The reports of those who have already tried it and have conscientiously followed the plan show tremendous success. Satisfied customers claim a variety of advantages, but the most widely mentioned ones are an increased zest for life and a feeling of well being. Because the body of every human varies in type and in build, so the benefits vary. There are claims of reduced waist lines, better posture, reduced mental tension, increased capacity for work and indeed life, the ability to sleep better, a better distribution of fat, increased self-confidence, more regular internal workings and an awakened desire to take part in active sport . . . these are and have been the most frequently mentioned benefits. There have also been some more surprising claims, such as increased bust measurements, a better sex life and even that a golf handicap has been reduced!! The mind boggles at these latter claims, but the theme is the same. The system works.

The Commando 7 is a series of seven exercises which are repeated a nominated number of times. Each exercise is aimed at a specific muscle group or area of the body and done together gives the whole body a conditioned work out. The men's exercises have been given three grades, but the women's only one. This has been done because the male body varies in physical fitness level much more than the female. As a rule the female maintains a higher standard of physical condition, because of the very nature of her natural metabolism and the normal physical activity of her life (housework, shopping, walking the baby, etc.). Hence, the woman tends to live longer than the man. None the less the Commando 7 exercises are important to both sexes and have been exclusively designed for both men and women.

There remains one question. When do I exercise? We offer no particular answer. Different times will suit different people. What is essential is that the exercises are done regularly each day. Psychologically it will be found easier to get into a routine and exercise at the same time each day. The exercise session is then made into a habit and is therefore much easier to accept. The favourite time is probably before breakfast, because there is less excuse at that time to put off the exercise period because of social or work commitments. Many will prefer the evening because the session clears the daily work and residual tension out of the system. On the other hand, those with a weight problem may prefer the lunch hour, because the exercise period can take the place of a large lunch and enable the subject to substitute a quick drink, a sandwich and a bowl of soup in order that he or she can do the daily schedule. It does not really matter when, but it does matter that you do your Commando 7 Exercises every day. If you make exercising a daily habit, then you will find it easier to complete the programme and get fit.

The exercise plan will achieve its aim if done in isolation, but will be even more effective if complemented by walking or running, when the opportunity occurs. After a couple of weeks on course, it is well worth the conscious effort to walk rather than take that bus or taxi. Gradually you will feel more like taking this sort of loco-motory exercise; walking up the stairs rather than taking the lift will present a challenge which you will want to take and you will feel all the better for it. There are hundreds of little things which can help the ultimate object—the physical efficiency of your body.

In this chapter we have given you the why, how and when of the Commando 7 Exercises. They were originally written for a television-viewing public in the North East of England and had to be quick, safe, effective and simple. No equipment could be used. It was therefore within these limitations that the exercises were designed, tested and published. The remarkable fact is that they really do provide a formula for the body to get fit. It is a formula which we give you to follow.

CHAPTER IV

THE TRAINER'S EXERCISE INSTRUCTIONS AND MEDICAL ADVICE

Safety and simplicity are two of the principles on which the Commando 7 Exercises programme has been based. There are, however, rules to be noted and certain medical factors to be known and understood by anyone starting to exercise. This is what is contained in this chapter.

Before giving suggested age brackets and specific rules, it is necessary to state that if you have not taken regular exercise for some considerable time, been physically inactive for two years, are very much over-weight, have suffered from a heart or respiratory condition or have recently been ill, then take care and consult a doctor before starting this or any exercise programme.

The golden rule, because of the different physical states of our various bodies, is that if you are in any doubt or if you can be classified, even loosely, in the terms of the broad description in the preceding paragraph, then consult your doctor. While the remainder of this chapter gives more detailed rules about age, physical condition and the actual exercise instructions, this rule must be overriding.

Having now given the formal medical warning, it can be stated with confidence that no medical problems were reported during the entire television showing of the exercises on provincial television in a densely populated area of the United Kingdom (Tyne Tees), nor has there since been any reported. Similarly, there have been no ill effects recorded or reported from the publication of the exercises in the *Sunday Times* or from Australia, where the exercise routines were also widely publicised. These facts are a clear recommendation of the proven safety of the exercises for people of all ages. This is an important factor.

The first restriction is a surprisingly loose one. When can the body start and when is it too old to start? First, we deal with the start mark. We set the lower age at about ten, although there can be no real lower age bracket which impinges on any safety problem over physical exercise. The body may simply not be ready to cope with the type of exercise detailed before about ten or eleven years of age, depending on the individual body development. There is little harm in any child trying the exercises and children can and will experiment with exercises. The Commando 7 Exercises are ideal for competition and experiment. The young body can try the exercises, but it is not at them that the programme is aimed.

The upper age limit is more difficult to assess. One of the original test subjects was a miner aged sixty-eight and he seemed to thrive on the exercises. The answer and the advice is therefore difficult to detail in exact terms. Little is really known about the ageing process. We all know that some people, because of the various factors discussed in previous chapters, appear to age more quickly than others. We all die at different ages. Nobody really knows the reasons, although the problem of growing old has been thought about since the beginning of time.

We believe that one of the real benefits of regular physical exercise is that it slows down the ageing process, because it increases the efficiency of the heart, lungs, muscles and joints of the body. It is a fair assumption that if a machine is well maintained, then it will last longer. The upper limit to starting the Commando 7 exercise programme is therefore hard to specify. A rough guide is as follows:

60 and above: Consult your doctor first. You will probably have more time for such activities as walking or light swimming and therefore may not need short daily exercise sessions. The Grade C exercises for men or those given for women could well be both beneficial and fun to do. Stop when you feel any discomfort, but double the number of days allowed.

Between 35 and 60: Your body should be capable of this sort of programme, but if in doubt consult a doctor first. Grade C should be tried by men nearing the sixty mark. Remember that the grossly overweight and chronically unfit should be careful.

Under 35: You have a problem if these exercises present any difficulty!

From this outline age guide you should now note the sort of medical conditions which should cause you to pause and take advice, if you happen to be a sufferer from any of them. Even then the doctor may allow you to proceed with confidence, *but ask him first*:

(a) Any heart or respiratory condition.
(b) High blood pressure.
(c) Any infectious disease.
(d) Gross obesity.
(e) Kidney or liver complaints.
(f) Diabetes.
(g) Anything which gives you pain.

There may be other medical conditions which may preclude an exercise programme and so anybody being treated by a doctor should naturally consult him before starting the exercise routines. Generally, and even for some of the conditions detailed above (note the number of top sportsmen who are diabetics!), a doctor will advise you that the sort of routine we suggest is safe or he will give you the scale to which you can participate. Few medical men will ever have to advise you to take NO exercise, although there are some conditions which preclude any exercise except mild walking. Exercise is, almost always, good news!

We can now move to the actual exercises themselves. The Commando 7 is a ten-week programme of short daily exercise sessions, which is designed to get the human body physically fit without the use of any apparatus or equipment. The plan is progressive and offers three grades for men and one for women. For men the B grade is the average grade. Each session has to be done once a day for one week. On completion of a week on the same set of exercises, the subject moves to the next week's exercises and repeats the programme. At Week 8 there is a test, also done each day, instead of the normal programme. For Weeks 9 and 10 you again follow the exercise routines. At the end of the tenth week you will be physically fitter and should both see and feel your progress.

One point to watch is that you do the exercises properly. The more you put into them the more the benefit to be gained. The second point is that you must take your time. A slowly worked programme is infinitely better than one which is rushed through. You can take a thirty-second rest at the end of each separate exercise group. Some people may well be aware that the early sessions take very little time; this is acknowledged, but this is a general programme which is aimed at the very wide spectrum of the population. Whatever you feel, keep to the progress chart and aim to get fit in the prescribed ten weeks.

To the problem posed by injury or sickness, if suffered during the programme, we suggest a simple rule of thumb. The same rule will apply if you happen to miss a session for some reason or other. The rule is that if you lose less than 48 hours, do the sessions you have missed and maintain your normal progress through the plan, ending it two days later than originally expected. For any longer period, go back a week for every two days lost.

The last pre-exercise instruction concerns the physical preparation. We believe that it is useful if the body is "loosened up" prior to actually tackling the first exercise of the day. Such a warm up can be as simple as this:

Stand with your feet apart and circle the arms, possibly doing swimming strokes in the air for a few seconds ... then bend forwards and backwards a few times ... now move very slowly to a crouch position and repeat two or three times ...

A very gentle running on the spot will complete a suitable "warm up". You can of course go for a short walk or climb up and down the stairs a few times; the principle is the same, to warm the body through and start the blood moving a little more swiftly than usual.

Most people require a positive aim if they are to achieve anything. A fitness programme is no exception. The athlete and the sportsman usually have an aim, the motivating factor is the stop watch, the tape measure or just the satisfaction of victory or doing well. For the average person, however, the aim of "getting fit", despite all the advantages which have been stated in this book, is an elusive aim at the start of the course.

It was to give an incentive and a progress check that we included a test in Week 8 of the course. The younger person can make this eighth-week test all the more interesting by trying to do the test before he starts the course and then do the test in Week 8 of the programme, just to see the difference, as well as feel it! The repetitions are increased as the weeks' programmes are changed and so for the exerciser the progress will be apparent by virtue of the fact that the next week's exercises can be completed.

Another way which can add interest is if you learn to take your pulse correctly, or can persuade anybody to take it for you just prior to taking vigorous exercise. You then take if after the exercise and at ten-minute intervals after that; you can see how long it takes you to return to a normal pulse rate. This can give you a pretty fair idea of your physical shape. The normal is round 72, but many people have pulses which are "normal" at different rates to that given as "normal". The shorter the recovery rate, generally speaking, the fitter you are. We hope that the progress will be evident enough without the necessity to have to continually test yourself, but pulse-taking can be fun!

We do not deal with diet in this chapter, because we are dealing with the instructions for actually participating in the programme. Your fuel intake (food and drink) and the subsequent maintenance of fitness are dealt with in Chapter VII. Suffice it to say at this stage that these exercises will help to burn off a bit of the excess fuel intake in your current diet, which otherwise might get deposited on your hips or add to your waistline. You may find that the weighing machine tells a tale, though no guarantee is given. The exerciser can, however, help by eating less of the obviously fattening foods.

The reader should now be ready to turn the page and start on Week 1. Before doing so, remember the medical warning. It must be clearly understood and if it is ignored, then the authors of this safe and effective exercise plan can take no responsibility. Admittedly the chances of any problems arising are negligible, because it is a tried and tested system, but this chapter has spelt out the rules. By obeying these rules and by following the exercise instructions, a physically safer future is within your grasp, through the Commando 7 Exercise Plan.

CHAPTER V

THE COMMANDO 7 EXERCISE ROUTINES FOR MEN

Week 1

1. *Half press ups*

From a standing position kneel down. Lean your body forward placing your hands in front of your shoulders and on the ground so that the hands can support your upper body. Now bend and stretch your arms, keeping the knees on the ground. **A15 B10 C6**

2. *Side bending*

From a standing position with hands at the sides bend the body from the waist, left then right, with the feet slightly apart. Reach down as far as you can, down the outside of your legs—you should be able to touch below the knee area. **A15 B10 C6**

3. *½ Squats*

From the standing position bend the knees to a semi-sitting position, raising the arms horizontally at the same time. Now return to the standing position, by straightening the knees and lowering the arms. **A15 B10 C6**

4. *Dorsal exercise*

Lie face down with hands clasped behind the back. Raise the trunk and legs off the ground, simultaneously. **A12 B8 C4**

5. *Burpees exercise*

From standing, stoop to the crouch position with hands on the floor. Then shoot the legs backwards to the front support position. Return to the crouch position and then stand up. This is a "burpee". **A10 B5 C2**

6. *Sit ups*

Lie on your back, then rise without use of your arms, almost to a sitting position. The hands must be able to touch the knee caps. Return to lying on the back. **A15 B10 C5**

7. *Spot running*

Run on the spot for ten paces, counting as the left foot touches the ground. On completion of ten paces, then do one ½ squat. **A4 B3 C1**

WEEK 1

Week 2

1. *Press ups*

Lie on the ground, face downwards. Place the palms of the hands underneath the shoulders. Now force the body off the ground until you are supporting the body weight with the arms and toes. This is the press up position. The arms are now bent and stretched allowing the chest to touch the ground lightly. This is one movement and is a press up. **A10 B5 C3**

2. *Side bending*

From a standing position with hands at the sides bend the body from the waist, left then right, with the feet slightly apart. Reach down as far as you can, down the outside of your legs—you should be able to touch below the knee area. **A20 B16 C8**

3. ½ *Squats*

From the standing position bend the knees to a semi-sitting position, raising the arms horizontally at the same time. Now return to the standing position, by straightening the knees and lowering the arms. **A20 B12 C8**

4. *Dorsal exercise*

Lie face down with hands clasped behind the back. Raise the trunk and legs off the ground, simultaneously. **A16 B10 C6**

5. *Burpees*

From standing, stoop to the crouch position with hands on the floor. Then shoot the legs backwards to the front support position. Return to the crouch position and then stand up. This is a "burpee". **A14 B8 C5**

6. *Sit ups*

Lie on your back, then rise without use of your arms, almost to a sitting position. The hands must be able to touch the knee caps. Return to lying on the back. **A20 B15 C8**

7. *Spot running*

Run on the spot for ten paces, counting as the left foot touches the ground. On completion of ten paces, then do one ½ squat. **A5 B4 C2**

34

WEEK 2

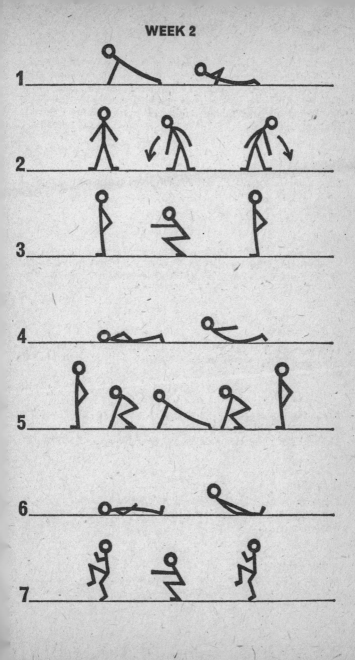

Week 3

1. *Press ups*

Lie on the ground, face downwards. Place the palms of the hands underneath the shoulders. Now force the body off the ground until you are supporting the body weight with the arms and toes. This is the press up position. The arms are now bent and stretched allowing the chest to touch the ground lightly. This is one movement and is a press up.   **A15 B10 C5**

2. *Side bending*

From a standing position, this time with opposite arm curling underneath armpit. Left then right.   **A25 B20 C10**

3. *½ Squats*

From the standing position bend the knees to a semi-sitting position, raising the arms horizontally at the same time. Now return to the standing position, by straightening the knees and lowering the arms.
                                                                    A25 B16 C10

4. *Dorsal exercise*

Lie face down with hands clasped behind the back. Raise the trunk and legs off the ground, simultaneously.   **A20 B12 C8**

5. *Burpees*

From standing, stoop to the crouch position with hands on the floor. Then shoot the legs backwards to the front support position. Return to the crouch position and then stand up.   **A18 B12 C6**

6. *Sit ups*

Lie on your back, this time with hands clasped behind the neck. A full sit up to the vertical position. You may need to bend your knees.   **A20 B10 C5**

7. *Spot running*

Run on the spot for ten paces, counting as the left foot touches the ground. On completion of ten paces, then do one ½ squat. **A6 B5 C3**

WEEK 3

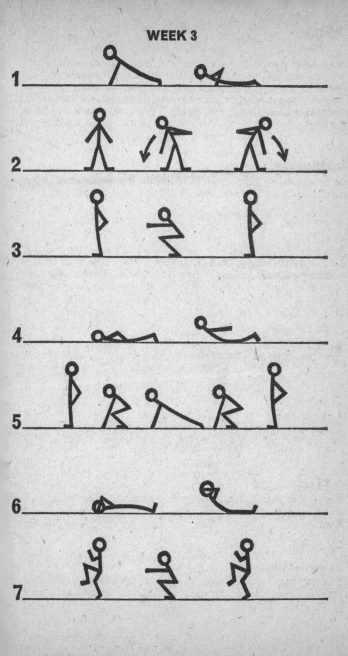

Week 4

1. *Press ups*

Lie on the ground, face downwards. Place the palms of the hands underneath the shoulders. Now force the body off the ground until you are supporting the body weight with the arms and toes. This is the press up position. The arms are now bent and stretched allowing the chest to touch the ground lightly. This is one movement and is a press up.   **A20 B15 C8**

2. *Side bends*

From standing position with feet astride. The opposite arm is now stretched over the head as you bend sideways, left then right.

A20 B14 C12

3. *½ Squats*

From the standing position bend the knees to a semi-sitting position, raising the arms horizontally at the same time. Now return to the standing position, by straightening the knees and lowering the arms.   **A30 B16 C12**

4. *Dorsal exercise*

Lie face down with hands clasped behind the back. Raise the trunk and legs off the ground, simultaneously.   **A25 B14 C10**

5. *Burpees*

From standing, stoop to the crouch position with hands on the floor. Then shoot the legs backwards to the front support position. Return to the crouch position and then stand up.   **A20 B14 C8**

6. *Sit ups*

From lying on back position, hands clasped behind the neck. Sit up to a vertical position. You may need to bend your knees.

A25 B15 C8

7. *Spot running*

Run on the spot for ten paces, counting as the left foot touches the ground. On completion of ten paces, then do one ½ squat. **A8 B6 C4**

WEEK 4

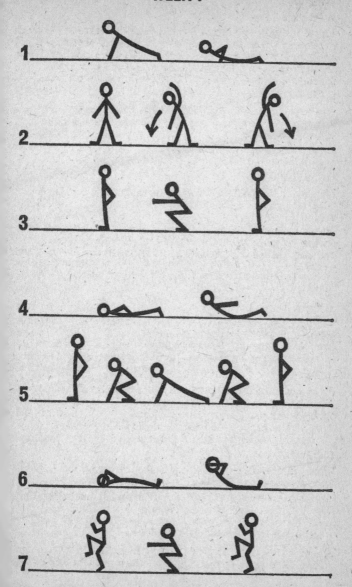

Week 5

1. Press ups

Perform 16 press ups from front support position as before. Then perform 4 inverted press ups. The same position but now with the hands turned inwards, so fingers are touching.   **A30 B20 C10**

2. Side bends

From standing position with feet astride. The opposite arm is now stretched over the head as you bend sideways, left then right.

A24 B18 C14

3. Squat jumps

From a standing position, drop to a $\frac{1}{2}$ squat position and then jump upwards, a foot or more off the floor.   **A15 B8 C4**

4. Dorsal exercise

Lie on the front as before but this time with hands touching the shoulders. Lift the trunk and legs off the ground and return to lying down.   **A20 B16 C8**

5. Burpees

From standing, stoop to the crouch position with hands on the floor. Then shoot the legs backwards to the front support position. Return to the crouch position and then stand up.   **A24 B16 C10**

6. Sit ups

From lying on back position, hands clasped behind the neck. Sit up to a vertical position and return to lying down.   **A30 B20 C10**

7. Spot running

Run on the spot for ten paces, counting as the left foot touches the ground. On completion of ten paces do a star stand from the crouch position. The star stand position is achieved with a slight jump from the crouch position. Your arms go upwards and apart, your legs go wide astride. The sequence is ten paces and one star jump.   **A6 B4 C4**

WEEK 5

Week 6

1. *Press ups*

Perform 18 press ups from front support position as before. Then perform 6 inverted press ups. The same position but now with the hands turned inwards, so fingers are touching. **A36 B24 C15**

2. *Side bends*

From standing position with feet astride. The opposite arm is now stretched over the head as you bend sideways, left then right.

A30 B22 C16

3. *Squat jumps*

From a standing position, drop to a $\frac{1}{2}$ squat position and then jump upwards, a foot or more off the floor. **A20 B10 C5**

4. *Dorsal exercise*

Lie on the front as before with hands touching the shoulders. Lift the chest and legs off the ground and return to lying down.

A22 B18 C10

5. *Burpees*

From standing, stoop to the crouch position with hands on the floor. Then shoot the legs backwards to the front support position. Return to the crouch position and then stand up. **A26 B18 C12**

6. *Sit ups*

From lying on back position, hands clasped behind the neck. Sit up to touch alternate knee with elbow (left elbow to right knee).

A36 B26 C16

7. *Spot running*

Run on the spot for ten paces, counting as the left foot touches the ground. On completion of ten paces do a star stand from the crouch position. The star stand position is achieved with a slight jump from the crouch position. Your arms go upwards and apart, your legs go wide astride. The sequence is ten paces and one star jump. **A7 B5 C5**

WEEK 6

Week 7

1. Press ups

Do 20 press ups from front support position. Then perform 5 hand clap press ups. For these, push upwards from front support position, clap hands and drop back to front support position.   **A30 B25 C15**

2. Side bends

From standing position with feet astride. The opposite arm is now stretched over the head as you bend sideways, left then right.

A34 B30 C20

3. Squat jumps

From a standing position, drop to a $\frac{1}{2}$ squat position and then jump upwards, a foot or more off the floor.   **A20 B16 C8**

4. Dorsal exercise

Lie on the front as before with hands touching the shoulders. Lift the trunk and legs off the ground and return to lying down.

A25 B20 C14

5. Double jump burpees

From standing position, take up a crouch position as for the ordinary burpee. Jump the legs backwards to front support position. Now jump both legs forward and backwards twice, before returning to the crouch position and standing up. This is a double jump burpee.

A20 B14 C8

6. Sit ups

From lying on back position, hands clasped behind the neck. Sit up to touch alternate knee with elbow (left elbow to right knee).

A45 B30 C18

7. Spot running

Run on the spot for ten paces, counting as the left foot touches the ground. Then do one star jump. The star jump is a leap from the crouch position with the hands in front to make a star in the air, with arms and legs wide apart and off the ground for a moment. The sequence is ten paces and one star jump.   **A8 B6 C6**

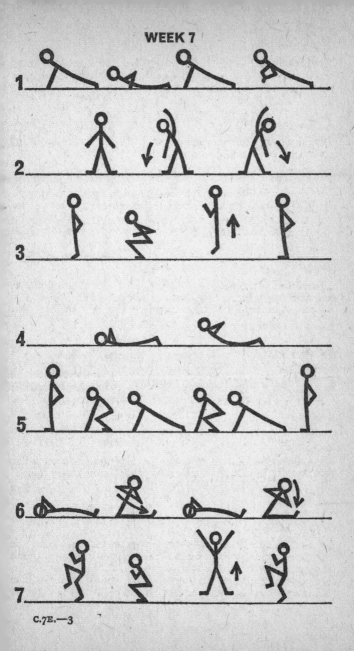

Week 8 TEST

Your Test Week

To check on your progress, the following tests should be followed each day:

1. *Press ups*
Press ups to personal maximum.

2. *Knee jumps*
To personal maximum in 30 seconds. A knee jump is a jump from a standing position. The knees jumped up together as high as possible.

3. *Sit ups*
Sit ups with hands clasped behind neck to personal maximum.

4. *Burpees*
Burpees to maximum, within 1 minute.
Allow two minutes rest after each exercise.

Performance chart	A Above average	B Average	C Below average
1. Press ups	20 or above	10–15	Under 9
2. Knee jumps	20 or above	10–15 in 30 seconds	Under 10
3. Sit ups	30 or above	10–25	Under 15
4. Burpees	30 or above	15–25 in 1 minute	Under 15

The points system has been devised as a performance guide for someone who was inactive before starting the Commando 7 course.

WEEK 8 TEST

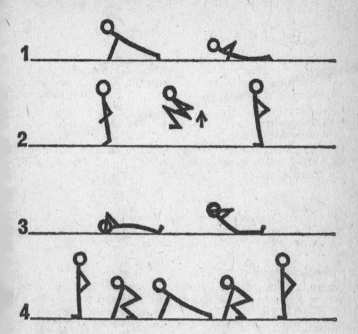

Week 9

1. *Press ups*

Do 22 press ups from front support position, plus 8 inverted press ups as described.   **A40 B30 C20**

2. *Side bending*

From standing with feet apart about 18 inches. Reach the arms above the head as far as possible. Bend from side to side, keeping the arms straight and moving the body in rhythm with the arms. Do the exercise both left and right.   **A35 B26 C20**

3. *Squat jumps*

From a standing position, drop to a $\frac{1}{2}$ squat position and then jump upwards, a foot or more off the floor.   **A25 B20 C16**

4. *Dorsal exercise*

Lie on the front with hands touching the shoulders. Lift the trunk and legs off the ground and return to lying down.   **A28 B16 C12**

5. *Double jump burpees*

From standing position, take up a crouch position as for the ordinary burpee. Jump the legs backwards to front support position. Now jump both legs forward and backwards twice, before returning to the crouch position and standing up. This is a double jump burpee.   **A24 B16 C12**

6. *Sit ups and leg raising*

30 sit ups from lying on the back, hands clasped behind the neck. Sit up to touch alternate knee with elbow (left elbow to right knee). Now add five leg raises. For the leg raises you keep the body on the ground and raise both legs about six inches off the floor. Hold this position for a count of five and then lower. The exercise is sit ups followed by five leg raises.   **A45 B35 C25**

7. *Spot running*

Spot running with 1 star jump at end of each sequence of ten paces.   **A10 B8 C7**

WEEK 9

1
2
3
4
5
6
7

Week 10

1. Press ups

25 press ups from front support position. Also perform 5 chest-slap press ups in the manner of the hand clap press up. Instead of clapping, touch chest and return to floor with hands. **A40 B30 C24**

2. Side bending

From standing with feet apart about 18 inches. Reach the arms above the head as far as possible. Bend from side to side, keeping the arms straight and moving the body in rhythm with the arms. Do the exercise both left and right. **A50 B40 C30**

3. Squat jumping

From a standing position, drop to a $\frac{1}{2}$ squat position and then jump upwards, a foot or more off the floor. **A30 B22 C20**

4. Dorsal exercise

Lying face downwards with the hands clasped behind neck. Lift the trunk and legs off the ground. **A30 B18 C14**

5. Double jump burpee

From standing position, take up a crouch position as for the ordinary burpee. Jump the legs backwards to front support position. Now jump both legs forward and backwards twice, before returning to the crouch position and standing up. **A30 B20 C14**

6. Sit ups

Sit ups, with hands clasped behind the neck. After 35 sit ups do 5 leg raises. You lie on the back and raise both legs off the ground holding the position for a count of five. **A60 B40 C30**

7. Spot running

Spot running with a star jump at the end of each sequence of ten paces. **A12 B10 C8**

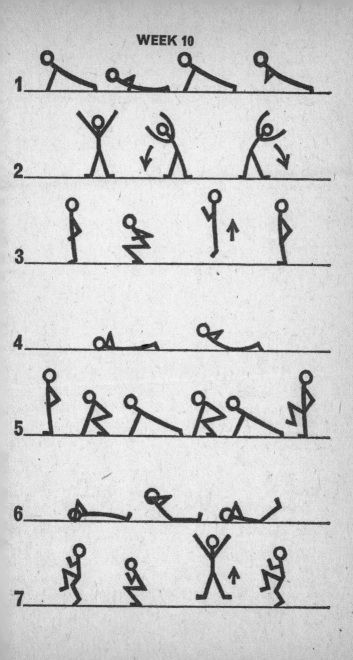

CHAPTER VI

THE COMMANDO 7 EXERCISES FOR WOMEN

Week 1

1. *Arm raising*

From the standing position place the feet apart and cross the wrists over the stomach. Keeping the arms straight swing them upwards and outwards and return.   **5 times**

2. *Leg raising*

Lie on the back and raise each leg alternately to as near a vertical position as possible.   **5 times**

3. *Side bending*

From a standing position, with feet slightly apart. Bend the body from the waist, left then right, reaching down the side of your leg as far as you can go.   **10 times**

4. *Dorsal exercise*

Lie face down, with hands grasped behind the back. Raise the trunk and legs off the ground simultaneously.   **5 times**

5. *Sit ups*

Lie on your back, then rise without use of your arms to a semi-sitting position. The hands must be able to cover the knee caps. Return to lying on the back.   **5 times**

6. *Burpees*

From standing, stoop to crouch position with hands on the floor. Then shoot legs backwards to press up position. Back to crouch position and then stand up. This is a "burpee".   **4 times**

7. *Spot running*

Run on the spot and keep count up to ten, using left leg as the marker as it touches the ground. Pause for five seconds and repeat. **3 times**

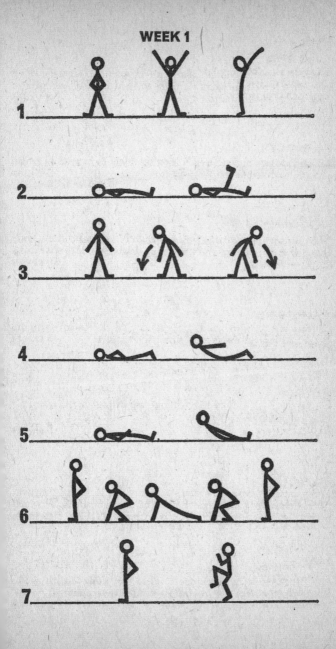

WEEK 1

Week 2

1. *Arm raising*

From the standing position place the feet apart and cross the wrists over the stomach. Keeping the arms straight swing them upwards and outwards and return.   **8 times**

2. *Leg raising*

Lie on the back and raise each leg alternately to as near a vertical position as possible.   **8 times**

3. *Side bending*

From a standing position, with feet slightly apart. Bend the body from the waist, left then right, reaching down the side of your leg as far as you can go.   **15 times**

4. *Dorsal exercise*

Lie face down, with hands grasped behind the back. Raise the trunk and legs off the ground simultaneously.   **6 times**

5. *Sit ups*

Lie on your back, then rise without use of your arms to a semi-sitting position. The hands must be able to cover the knee caps. Return to lying on the back.   **8 times**

6. *Burpees*

From standing, stoop to crouch position with hands on the floor. Then shoot legs backwards to press up position. Back to crouch position and then stand up. This is a "burpee".   **8 times**

7. *Spot running*

Run on the spot and keep count up to ten, using left leg as the marker as it touches the ground. Pause for five seconds and repeat.   **4 times**

WEEK 2

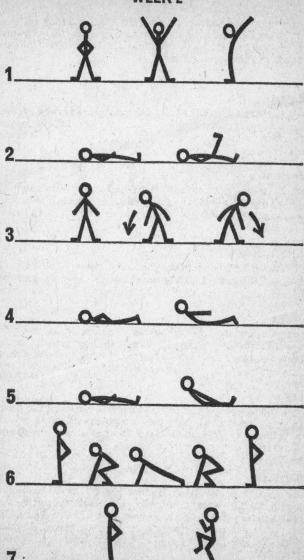

Week 3

1. *Arm raising*

From the standing position place the feet apart and cross the wrists over the stomach. Keeping the arms straight swing them upwards and outwards and return, but this time raise the heels and push the chest out as you raise the arms. **10 times**

2. *Leg raising*

Lie on the back and raise each leg alternately to as near a vertical position as possible, but this time count 1 2 3 4 5 as the leg goes to the vertical position. **8 times**

3. *Side bending*

From a standing position, with feet slightly apart with hands on shoulders. Bend the body from the waist, left then right, reaching down the side of your leg as far as you can go. **15 times**

4. *Dorsal exercise*

Lie face down, with hands grasped behind the back. Raise the trunk and legs off the ground simultaneously. **7 times**

5. *Sit ups*

Lie on your back, then rise without use of your arms to a semi-sitting position. The hands must be able to cover the knee caps. Return to lying on the back. **10 times**

6. *Burpees*

From standing, stoop to crouch position with hands on the floor. Then shoot legs backwards to press up position. Back to crouch position and then stand up. This is a "burpee". **9 times**

7. *Spot running*

Spot running with alternate half squat. You run as before, on the spot, counting the paces as the left foot touches the ground. At the end of ten paces you go into a half crouching position, called a half squat. Raise your arms horizontally as you get into the half squat position. The standing up position is resumed before starting the next sequence. **3 times**

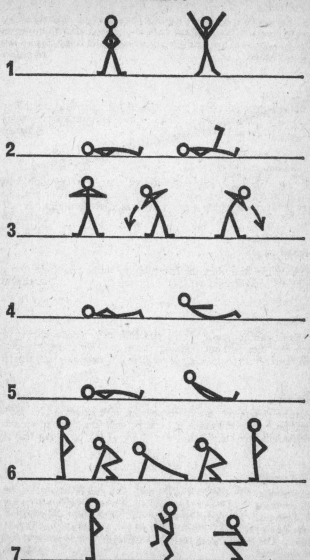

Week 4

1. *Arm raising*

From the standing position place the feet apart and cross the wrists over the stomach. Keeping the arms straight swing them upwards. When the arms are up, jerk them backwards and bring them down on the rebound.　　　　　　　　　　　　　　　　　**10 times**

2. *Leg raising*

From the lying on the back position, both legs are raised together to the vertical position, to the count of five. If in difficulty, stretch your arms outwards.　　　　　　　　　　　　　　　　**5 times**

3. *Side bending*

Standing with feet astride and with both hands on the shoulders. Bend from side to side, with one hand on the shoulder and the opposite arm stretching over the head. Left then right is one exercise.　　　　　　　　　　　　　　　　　　**20 times**

4. *Dorsal exercise*

Lie face down and place the hands on the shoulders. Raise upper trunk and legs off the floor.　　　　　　　　　　　　**8 times**

5. *Toe touching*

From the standing position with feet about 18 inches apart try to touch the toes without bending the knees. Do the movement slowly and return to standing position, feet astride.　　**14 times**

6. *Burpees*

From standing, stoop to crouch position with hands on the floor. Then shoot legs backwards to press up position. Back to crouch position and then stand up.　　　　　　　　　　　**10 times**

7. *Spot running*

Spot running with alternate half squat. You run as before, on the spot, counting the paces as the left foot touches the ground. At the end of ten paces you go into a half crouching position, called a half squat. Raise your arms horizontally as you get into the half squat position. The standing up position is resumed before starting the next sequence.　　　　　　　　　　　　　　　**4 times**

WEEK 4

Week 5

1. Arm raising

From the standing position place feet apart and cross the wrists over the stomach. Keeping the arms straight swing them upwards. When the arms are up, jerk them backwards and bring them down on the rebound.   **12 times**

2. Leg raising

From the lying on the back position, both legs are raised together to the vertical position, to the count of five. If in difficulty, stretch your arms outwards.   **8 times**

3. Side bending

Standing with feet astride and with both hands on the shoulders. Bend from side to side, with one hand on the shoulder and the opposite arm stretching over the head. Left then right is one exercise.   **24 times**

4. Dorsal exercise

Lie face down and place hands on the shoulders. Raise upper trunk and legs off the floor and hold for a slow count of three.   **8 times**

5. Toe touching

From the standing position with feet about 18 inches apart try to touch the toes without bending the knees but this time with both hands attempting to touch the left foot, then stand up. Then attempt to touch the right foot, then stand up.   **8 times**

6. Burpees

From standing, stoop to crouch position with hands on the floor. Then shoot legs backwards to press up position. Back to crouch position and then stand up.   **11 times**

7. Spot running

Spot running with alternate half squat. You run as before, on the spot. Counting the paces as the left foot touches the ground. At the end of ten paces you go into a half crouching position, called a half squat. Raise your arms horizontally as you get into the half squat position. The standing up position is resumed before starting the next sequence.   **4 times**

WEEK 5

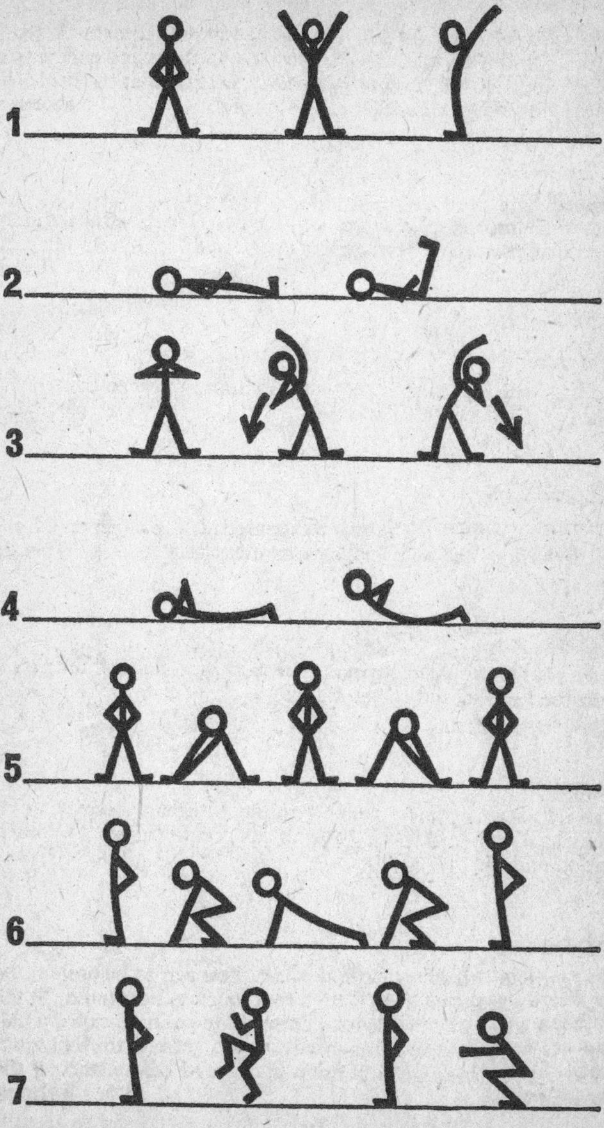

Week 6

1. Arm stretching

Stand with feet wide astride and the hands stretched out in front of you, parallel to the ground. Now move the arms wide apart and rebound to the forward position, with the arms stretched straight out in front parallel to the ground.   **16 times**

2. Leg raising

From the lying on the back position, both legs are raised together to the vertical position, to the count of five. If in difficulty, stretch your arms outwards.   **10 times**

3. Side bending

Standing with feet astride and with both arms clasped behind the neck. Now bend from side to side.   **24 times**

4. Dorsal exercise

Lie face down and place hands on shoulders. Raise upper trunk and legs off the floor and hold for a slow count of four.   **8 times**

5. Sit ups

Lie on your back with arms in neck rest position (behind the neck). Sit to the vertical and return to lying down.   **12 times**

6. Burpees

From standing, stoop to crouch position with hands on the floor. Then shoot legs backwards to press up position. Back to crouch position and then stand up.   **10 times**

7. Spot running

Spot running with alternate half squat. You run as before, on the spot. Counting the paces as the left foot touches the ground. At the end of ten paces you go into a half crouching position, called a half squat. Raise your arms horizontally as you get into the half squat position. The standing up position is resumed before starting the next sequence.   **6 times**

WEEK 6

Week 7

1. *Arm stretching*

With the arms bent across the chest at shoulder height, feet apart no more than 18 inches. Keeping the arms up, throw back as far as possible. Hold that position and press back before returning to the original position with the arms across the chest. **16 times**

2. *Leg raising*

This time while lying on the back, raise both legs together six inches off the ground and hold for a slow count of three and return to floor. **10 times**

3. *Side bending*

Standing with feet astride and with both arms stretched up over the head. Move sideways 5 to left, 5 to right. **10 times**

4. *Dorsal exercise*

This time lie on the front with hands grasped behind the neck. Lift trunk off the ground with legs and hold for a count of three seconds. **8 times**

5. *Sit ups*

Lie on your back with arms in neck rest position (behind the neck) Sit up to the vertical and return to lying down. **12 times**

6. *Burpees*

From standing, stoop to crouch position with hands on the floor. Then shoot legs backwards to press up position. Back to crouch position and then stand up. **14 times**

7. *Spot running*

Spot running with alternate half squat. You run as before, on the spot. Counting the paces as the left foot touches the ground. At the end of ten paces you go into a half crouching position, called a half squat. Raise your arms horizontally as you get to the half squat position. The standing up position is resumed before starting the next sequence. **6 times**

WEEK 7

1

2

3

4

5

6

7

Week 8 TEST

This test is designed to see how you have progressed and yet continue the work programme of ten weeks.

Do the tests each day, with two minutes' rest between each exercise sequence.

1. *Sit ups*

Lying down, with hands on the ground, sit up to where the hands can cover the knee caps and return. Try to match the score below.

2. *Burpees*

Standing, move to crouch position, shoot legs to rear and the press up position, return to the crouch position and then stand up. Try to match the score below.

3. ½ *Squats*

From standing position. Bend knees and raise both hands vertically out in front parallel with the ground. Try to match the score below.

Test Scores

1. *Sit ups* without pausing

Average 10–20. Above average 20 and above. Below average or you have not been following the exercise programme properly, under 10.

2. *Burpees* without pausing

Average 10–15 in a minute.
Above average over 15 in a minute.
Below average under 10 in a minute.

3. ½ *Squats* without pausing

Average 10–16.
Above average over 16.
Below average under 10.

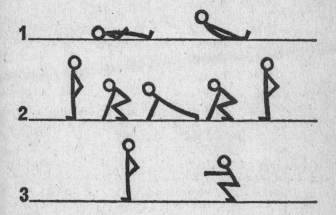

Week 9

1. *Arm stretching*

With the arms bent across the chest at shoulder height, feet apart no more than 18 inches. Keeping the arms up, throw back as far a possible. Hold that position and press back before returning to the original position with the arms across the chest.   **25 times**

2. *Leg raising*

Lying on the back, now lift both legs six inches off the floor, bend to bunched up position, stretch and lower.   **10 times**

3. *Side bending*

This time with hands clasped behind the neck. Feet 18 inches apart Bend sideways. Hold downward position to count of 5 seconds and return to upright position. Left then right.   **20 times**

4. *Dorsal exercise*

This time lie on the front with hands grasped behind the neck. Lif trunk off the ground with legs and hold for a count of five seconds   **8 times**

5. *Trunk circling*

Stand with the hands on the hips. Perform trunk circling leftward and then to the right. Do not move the feet which should be astride.   **10 times**

6. *Leg jumping*

From the front support position. Jump alternate legs forward and backwards.   **30 times**

7. *Spot running*

Spot running with alternate half squat. You run as before, on the spot. Counting the paces as the left foot touches the ground. At the end of ten paces you go into a half crouching position, called a half squat. Raise your arms horizontally as you get into the half squat position. The standing up position is resumed before starting the next sequence.   **8 times**

WEEK 9

Week 10

1. Rhythm press ups

Go into a kneeling position, bent forward so that the main weight of the body is taken by the arms. From this position stretch the body rhythmically forward so the chin touches the floor and return to sitting on the heels. Repeat.   **10 times**

2. Sit ups

This time lie on back with hands clasped behind the neck. Sit up and touch opposite knee with the elbow e.g. right elbow to left knee. 6 times each knee. You may bend your knees if you wish. **12 times**

3. Side bending

With arms raised in a reaching position above the head. Bend from side to side and hold for five seconds in side bend position. Ten bends each way.   **20 times**

4. Dorsal exercise

This time with hands clasped behind the neck, raise the upper trunk and alternate leg off the floor. Ten lifts of each leg. **20 times**

5. Bending exercise

Stand with the feet apart about eighteen inches. Lower the trunk keeping the knees straight. With up and down motions touch the ground in front of the legs, between the feet and behind the feet. Return to standing up, feet astride position.   **20 times**

6. Leg jumping

Front support position. As for press ups. Jump both legs forward and backwards together.   **10 times**

7. Spot running

Spot running and at the end of the ten pace series, do one burpee.
                    6 times

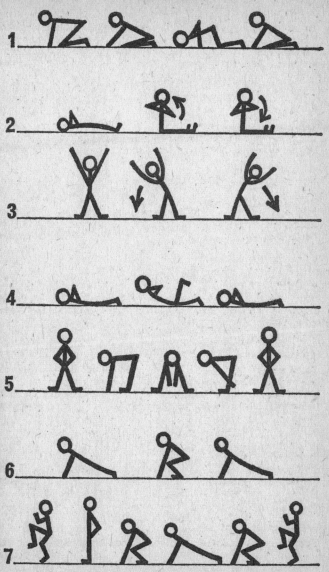

CHAPTER VII

MAINTAINING PHYSICAL FITNESS

Maintaining physical fitness is a problem which can be easily solved if you really wish to keep fit. We do not advise any strict rules which would clearly be impractical for the average citizen to obey, but suggest certain guidelines which can be reasonably applied to everyday living. The two main principles are regular exercise and sensible eating.

Before considering the subject of exactly what regular exercise you should take, it is worth reviewing your fuel, or food, intake. The most damaging aspect about food is that we all tend, without necessarily being conscious of it, to over-eat. The food, or fuel, which is excess to the body's requirements is not used or "burnt off" and will therefore turn into body fat. This fat is extra and unnatural weight which can make even the smallest physical task seem like hard work and places undue pressure of work on the ill-prepared and probably inefficient heart. Frequently it is this sort of situation which makes the body receptive to heart disease and the early grave.

There are many different views about the food substances we eat in the Western world today. Modern methods of food preparation and production have combined with various economic factors to change the basic content and nutritional value of much that is eaten by the human of today. The excessive quantities of sugar, fats and salt in the average person's diet are thought to be dangerous to health in the long term. The stomach is frequently filled and yet the body's nutritional needs are not necessarily met. The result is an unhealthy equation in which too much food combines with too little nutritional value and is multipled in danger by lack of exercise.

There is a bewildering collection of literature available on diet and it is difficult to summarize all this advice and instruction to give a clear direction for you to follow. Knowledge of nutrition is interpreted in many different ways and personal circumstances vary so much throughout society that it would be unwise for us to express firm views. All that we can do is to give the known principles of nutrition and offer advice based on the facts.

First, man eats to build, maintain and repair the protoplasm that makes up the body. Second, he eats to provide energy which is used either to keep the body warm or for physical work. Food must therefore provide the essential ingredients for the maintenance, work and heating of the body. The foods we eat can therefore be broadly classified into the body building, energy providing and the protective.

Protein is the main food for body building and it is for this reason that the "heavy" athletes such as shot putters, discus throwers and weight lifters eat a lot of protein. Energy can be obtained from all the main food types, but carbohydrates and fats are the main source. The final group are the protective foods and these are the substances called vitamins. The right combination of proteins, carbohydrates, fats and vitamins make up the balanced diet.

Examples of Food Classifications

A. *Energy-giving food*

Carbohydrates		Fats
Fruit		Nuts
Leaves		Seeds
Roots		Cooking fats
Jams	Sugar	Peanut butter
Treacles		Milk fat
Syrups		Butter
Sweets		Cheese
		Suet
Grain		Lard
Seeds		Fish oil
Roots		
Wheat	Starch	
Potatoes		
Bread		
Cakes		
Cereals		

Chops	—	Glucose
Milk	—	Lactose
Honey	—	Sucrose
Steaks	—	Glycogen

B. *Body-building food*

Proteins

All meat and poultry
Fish
Milk
Eggs
Roe
Cheese

Leaves
Seeds
Roots
Wheat } 2nd class
Bread
Potatoes

C. *Protective food*

Vitamins A. Spinach, Kale, Carrots, Peas, Beans, Animal
            Liver, Fish, Milk, Egg yolk, Butter, Cream.
       B. Rice, Wheat, Peas, Nuts, Yeast, Liver, Bacon,
            Lean meat, Milk, Eggs, Cheese.
       C. Greens, Citrus fruits, Tomatoes, Rosehips,
            Peas, Potatoes, Meat, Liver, Milk.
       D. Fish liver (Cod liver oil), Milk, Butter, Cream,
            Cheese, small amounts in vegetables, fruit and
            cereals.
       E. Lettuce, Peas, Wheat germ, small quantities
            in Meat, Milk, Cream, Butter.
       K. Spinach, Kale, Cabbage, Cauliflower,
            Cereals, Tomatoes, Carrots, Potatoes.

Note: Cocoa contains all known vitamins.

From this brief summary of basic nutritional principles we can understand why your eating habits are important to your physical condition. Although we do not intend to give a formally listed diet in our plan for physical fitness, we do suggest you avoid an excess of any food, but particularly the carbohydrate type. We think it is helpful for you to be aware of the nutritional value of your menu and think it relevant to the maintenance of fitness. The right sort of food is important to health, but it is not the main factor. The person who takes regular exercise can afford to be a little more careless in his eating habits because he will expend more energy and burn up the excess carbohydrates more easily. The maintenance of physical fitness becomes easier by sensible eating just as surely as a car will run on good quality petrol and the right sort of oil. It is, however, the actual maintenance of physical fitness to which we now turn.

Some people have reported that they have maintained a good standard of fitness just by continuing with the Commando 7 programme. This seems too repetitive to others who have continued the exercises but adapted the given repetitions. One such person reports that by doing this he managed to reduce his waist from 42 inches to 33 inches, with no conscious effort to diet! We believe that it is possible to retain a certain level of fitness by doing a Commando 7 schedule from after Week 5, daily, or almost daily, once you have completed the course. The occasional test taken from Week 8 of the course is good to check that your standards have not slipped. The Commando 7 routines are, however, a course of exercises which aims to get you fit, rather than keep you fit.

Exercise should be fun as well as beneficial and we have printed some similar exercise routines to the Commando 7 in the Maintenance Routines. The first are the full routines published by the *Sunday Times* as a Wall Chart of exercises and the second is a fitness maintenance exercise routine published in the same newspaper to complete the Commando 7 series. You can select your daily exercise routine from these maintenance sessions and use them with those from the Commando 7 series. Variety always adds interest to the necessary ritual of exercising the body.

The best way of maintaining physical fitness is always by natural movement or locomotory exercise. If you have, or can make, the time, then a regular walk, run or active game will provide the right sort of physical exercise and therefore body maintenance. The selected activity should demand real energy. Regrettably, the weekly round of golf hardly meets this requirement because it is so slow and the heart is rarely required to work above the level demanded of a slow walk. It is, however, much better than nothing.

The sort of activities in which you can usefully participate are: running, walking, swimming, cycling, squash, tennis, badminton, raquets, football, hockey, rugby football, netball, rounders, ski-ing, skating, basketball, judo and many similar sports. Obviously there are a host of other sports which could be listed and any sport which offers you a chance to get a sweat up and speeds the heart pumping blood around the body is a good exercise. The criterion is that energy is needed and that your body is physically worked. Some sports, like boxing, are only suitable for the very young or exceptionally fit. Others like rugby football and football have an effective age barrier because of the injury hazard over about thirty, whereas others can be enjoyed until late in life with comparative safety, provided they are played regularly.

For those who are not able to take part in sport, there are several ways of helping the body by exercising which occur during the average day. Every house has, for instance, a staircase and a regular series of stair climbing will soon raise the average pulse beat. The office will boast a long staircase and ten minutes a day going for a climb could well be a valuable type of exercise. Another simple form of exercise is "step ups" on a chair. A few series of twenty and the pulse will positively race!

For the unlucky ones who have few facilities available, the imagination has to be used. We advise you to positively look for exercise opportunities. A brisk walk round the block, a short run, a stair climb . . . the opportunities are often available if only they are recognised and accepted.

The next chapter gives some charts on fitness maintenance ideas, to which sensible eating habits can be usefully added. Exercise has to be frequent and regular. Recognition of these principles and the reader has a comprehensive recipe for a healthy life.

Food and Drink and Life

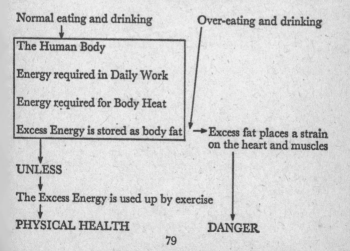

Normal eating and drinking   Over-eating and drinking

The Human Body

Energy required in Daily Work

Energy required for Body Heat

Excess Energy is stored as body fat → Excess fat places a strain on the heart and muscles

UNLESS

The Excess Energy is used up by exercise

PHYSICAL HEALTH   DANGER

CHAPTER VIII

FITNESS MAINTENANCE ROUTINES

1. PRESS UPS: 20 press ups from front support position, 5 hand clap press ups and 5 chest slap press ups. Total 30.

2. TRUNK CIRCLING: Stand with feet comfortably apart with hands placed on hips, circle the body in a 360-degree arc 8 times to the left and 8 times to the right. Total 16.

3. ASTRIDE JUMPS: With your hands on your hips, jump the feet apart and together rhythmically. This counts 1. Do 20.

4. BACK STRETCHING: Stand with back to wall, 18 inches away, with feet apart. Stretch arms backwards and up to touch wall above head, then forwards and down. 10 times.

5. BURPEES: From standing, stoop to crouched position with hands on the floor. Shoot the legs backwards to the push-up position, return to the crouch position and stand up. This is 1 burpee, repeat 20 times.

6. SIT UPS: Lie on back with hands clasped behind neck. Sit up to the vertical position. 30 times.

7. SPOT RUNNING: Run on the spot for 1 minute. Half-squat every 10 paces.

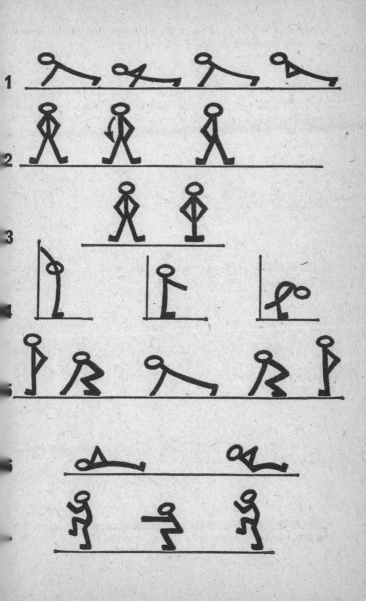

1. ARM CIRCLING: Stand with feet comfortably apart, arms stretched out sideways circle the arms forward 10 times, backwards 10 times. Total 20.

2. TRUNK CIRCLING: Stand with feet comfortably apart with hands placed on hips, the body in a 360-degree arc 10 times to the left and 10 times to the right. Total 20.

3. SIT UPS: Lie on back with hands clasped behind neck. Sit up to vertical position. 30 times.

4. SITTING TOE-TOUCHING: Sitting astride, touch each foot with both hands 10 times. Total 20.

5. STANDING STRAIGHT ARM-PRESSING: Hold out arms in front, palms facing. Press hands together with maximum effort for count of 5, keeping arms as straight as possible. Relax and repeat. 5 times.

6. STANDING TOE-TOUCHING: Feet comfortably apart, bend and attempt to touch each foot with both hands. Total 15.

7. ASTRIDE JUMPS: With your hands on your hips, jump the feet apart and together rhythmically. Total 20.

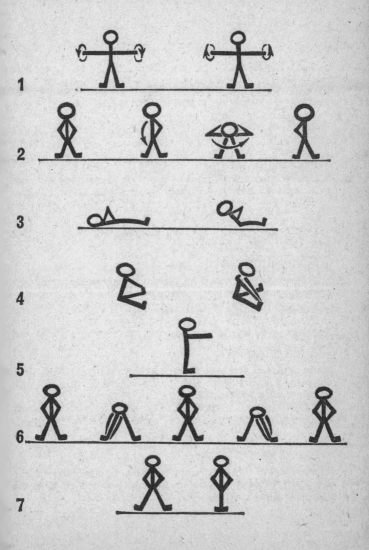

1. HEAD CIRCLING

Stand erect, feet comfortably apart, hands on hips. Pull chin in, circle head 10 times in one direction, then 10 times in other direction.

2. ARM CIRCLING

Stand erect, feet apart. Circle both arms simultaneously like propellers 10 times, then 10 times in reverse direction.

3. TRUNK TWISTING

Stand erect, feet apart, arms loosely by sides. Turn trunk and head to left and then to right. Repeat this whole movement left and right, 10 times.

4. TOE TOUCHING

Stand erect, feet apart. Bend down to touch toes, keeping legs straight if possible. Return to upright position. Repeat 10 times.

5. KNEE CLASPING

Stand erect, feet apart. Bend one knee upwards and pull it vigorously into your chest with both hands. Same with other knee and repeat 10 times with each knee.

6. ANKLE ROTATING

Sit on floor with one leg straight. Bend other leg over the straight leg, hold the foot of the bent leg and turn ankle as far as it will comfortably go in a circular movement. 10 times each ankle.

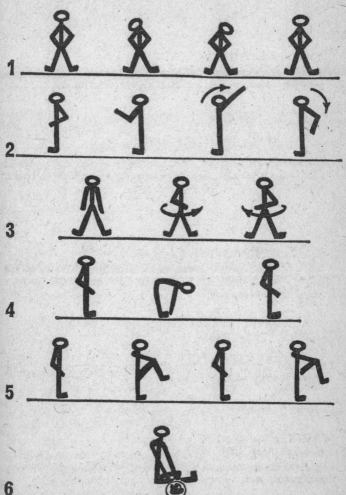

1. HALF PUSH UPS

Lie facing floor. With palms flat, push up till arms are straight, knees remaining on floor. Return to lying flat and repeat 10 times.

2. SITTING TOE TOUCHING

Sit with legs straight and apart, stretch right hand to touch left toe, then left hand to right toe. Repeat whole movement 30 times rhythmically.

3. SIT UPS

Lie on back. Rise without use of arms to near sitting position. Hands must touch kneecaps. Return to lying. Repeat 15 times.

4. SIDE BENDING

Stand with feet comfortably apart, hands on hips. Bend body from waist, reaching down as far as you can, first on left side, then on right. 20 times each side.

5. LEG RAISING

Lie on back and raise each leg alternately to the vertical. 20 times each leg.

6. SPOT RUNNING

Run on spot counting as right foot touches the floor. 100 paces in 1 minute.

1
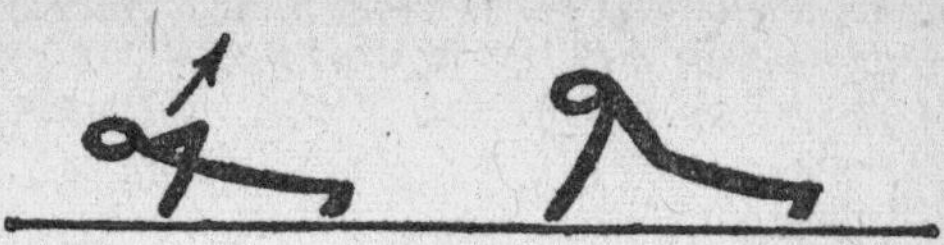

2

3

4
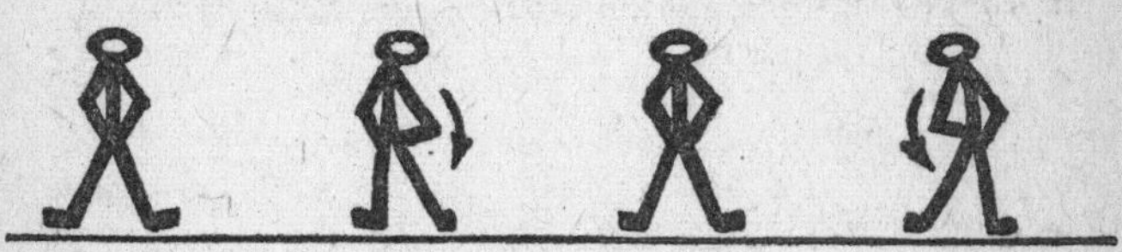

5
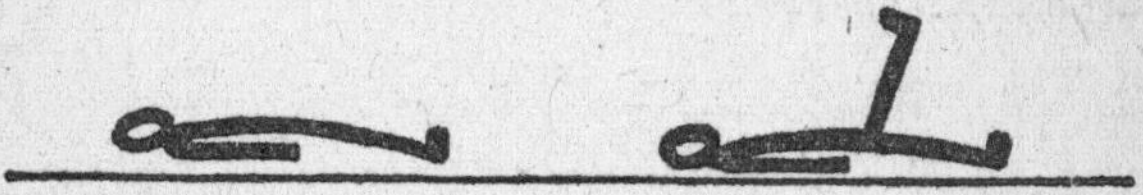

6

1. ARM RAISING

Stand with feet comfortably apart, cross wrists over stomach. Keeping arms straight, swing them upwards and outwards and return 20 times.

2. SIDE BENDING

Stand with feet comfortably apart, hands on hips. Bend body from waist, reaching down as far as you can, first on left side, then on right. 15 times each side.

3. SIT UPS

Lie on back. Rise without use of arms to near sitting position. Hands must touch kneecaps. Return to lying. Repeat 15 times.

4. SITTING TOE TOUCHING

Sit with legs straight and apart, stretch right hand to touch left toe, then left hand to right toe. Repeat whole movement 10 times rhythmically.

5. ASTRIDE JUMPS

With hands on hips, jump feet apart and then together again, repeating whole movement 30 times rhythmically.

6. SPOT RUNNING

Run on spot, counting as right foot touches floor. 40 paces.

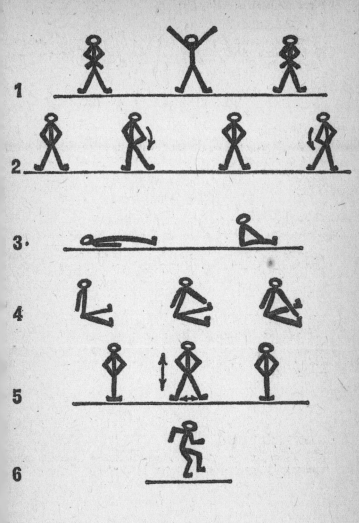

1

2

3.

4

5

6

1. PUSH UPS

Lie facing floor. With palms flat, push up till arms are straight and body is straight, supported on hands and toes. This time do not return to lying flat—just allow the chest to touch the floor lightly. Do as many as you can up to 20.

2. SIT UPS

Lie on back, hands clasped behind neck. Sit up to vertical position bending knees if necessary. 30 times.

3. DORSAL SWING

Stand with feet wide apart, hands by your sides, with back 12 inches away from wall. Touch wall between legs, then swing up to touch wall above head. 20 times.

4. LEG RAISING

Lie on back. Raise both legs to the vertical, then lower them slowly to floor. 15 times.

5. SKIP JUMPS

Stand with feet together, hands by sides. Spring up and down off the balls of your feet, 30 times. Repeat 30 times more, skipping with one foot forwards, other backwards, alternately.

6. BURPEES

From standing, crouch with hands on floor, then shoot legs backwards to the push-up position. Return to crouch and then stand up. This is one burpee. Repeat 15 times.

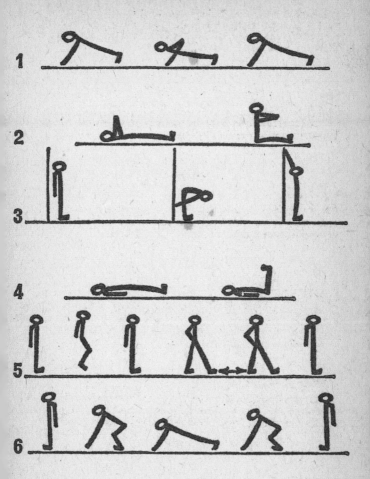

1. FREE STANDING SWIM

Stand with feet comfortably apart and swim the crawl, breast-stroke and back stroke. 20 of each.

2. TRUNK ROTATING

Stand with feet comfortably apart, arms stretched up above head. Make a circle with arms and trunk, brushing floor with hands in front at lowest point of movement. 10 times to left, 10 times to right.

3. SIT UPS

Lie on back, rise without use of arms to near sitting position. Hands must touch kneecaps. Return to lying. 20 times.

4. LEG RAISING

Lie on back. Raise both legs to the vertical, then lower them slowly (to count of 10) to floor. 10 times.

5. SKIP JUMPS

Stand with feet together, hands by sides. Spring up and down off the balls of your feet, 30 times. Repeat 30 times more, skipping with one foot forwards, other backwards alternately.

6. SPOT RUNNING

Run on spot for 1 minute.

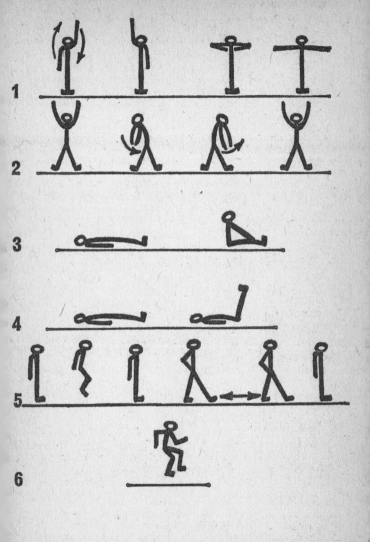

Fitness Maintenance Activities

Fitness maintenance activities are listed below in broad groupings as to their general classification. No attempt has been made to state that one particular grouping is necessarily of more value than another, although group A is probably of the most value to you physically, but will often require time and facilities which are not available. Group B can provide good exercise but we look upon them as a weaker method of exercise because they are often slow moving and do not guarantee the body a vigorous work out. Group C is a mixture of methods of exercising, some of which provide really heavy exercise and some of which are initiative methods of taking exercises. Group D is the Commando 7 Tables and the Fitness Maintenance Tables listed in this book.

Group A

Running—15 minutes plus
Brisk walking—30 minutes plus
Swimming—15 minutes plus
Cycling—15 minutes plus
Rowing
Skating
Football
Rugby Football and Rugby League
Hockey
Lacrosse
Basketball
Water Polo
Netball
Gymnastics

Squash
Badminton
Tennis
Fives
Handball
Raquets
Ice Hockey
Volleyball
Fencing
Judo
Wrestling
Ski-ing
Climbing
plus any similar activity

Group B

Baseball
Cricket
Golf
Gardening
Normal Walking (e.g. the dog)
Dancing

Group C

Circuit training
Weight training
Cycling machine
Rowing machine
Stair climbing—example: ten steps, climb up and down 3 times, pause for 30 seconds and repeat for 15 minutes.
Chair stepping—example: do 30 step ups to normal chair, pause for 30 seconds and repeat.

Group D
Any Commando 7 Table
Any of the Fitness Maintenance Tables

Fitness Maintenance Plan

Try to take exercise four times a week, with a minimum of three times. From the outline groupings in the list of Fitness Maintenance Activities you can create your own Fitness Maintenance Plan.

Example A. Men	*Week 1*	*Week 2*	*Week 3*	*Week 4*
Monday				
Tuesday	D	D	C	A
Wednesday				
Thursday	C	D	D	D
Friday				
Saturday	A	A	A	B
Sunday	B	B	A	A

The opportunity to exercise should certainly be taken on both week-end days because there will probably be the time available.

Example B. Women	*Week 1*	*Week 2*	*Week 3*	*Week 4*
Monday	D	A	D	A
Tuesday				
Wednesday	A	D	D	C
Thursday				
Friday	D	B	A	D
Saturday		A		A
Sunday	B		B	

Women will generally have more opportunity to exercise during week days than men and therefore exercise sessions at the week-end have not been emphasised.

It should be noted that should you have the time available to get in a Group A exercise then this is always acceptable in the maintenance of your physical fitness.

CHAPTER IX

SUPER FITNESS

The next step from being physically fit is not within the grasp of the average human. It is not, in fact, a necessary step, because it is enough just to be fit. It is sufficient for most of us to live life with an efficient and well-maintained body, the kernel of which is a healthy and strong heart. The realms of "super fitness" offer the extra and tangible challenge only for those who are young enough to aspire to excellence in sport, endurance or physical achievement.

The fact that the human has run at nearly 27 mph, jumped over 29 feet in length and over $7\frac{1}{2}$ feet in height, gives some indication of the possibilities which the super-fit body offers. It is, of course, wrong to pretend that these absolute peaks are within the human grasp because they are not. We all possess bodies with certain characteristics and qualities, some of which have greater physical potential than others. To the superb human specimen, hard work, dedication and technique can be combined to produce a person capable of great physical feats. Most of us have neither the time, the body nor the interest to realistically aspire to gold medal standards. There is, none the less, a clear message to be drawn from the top athlete in whatever field and that is that the body obviously responds to exercise. The body also shows remarkable resilience to hard physical work. This is particularly true of the younger person. There is a great store of untapped potential in most young bodies which regular and vigorous exercise will release. It is to those younger men to which this chapter is addressed, although it will interest the inquisitive from the ranks of those who are either too old, or hail from the weaker sex.

Nowhere is the response to exercise more apparent than in the Services where bodies which are normal for our modern society often "join up" in a pretty poor physical condition. The authors have personally seen some quite incredible improvements in physical capacity take place when these same bodies have been subjected to a disciplined physical training programme, that is, regular, progressive and vigorous. Admittedly the recruit has the motivating factor of wanting to be fit enough to join one of the world's elite fighting forces, the Royal Marines Commandos, but the fact is that the majority achieve their aim in a comparatively short time. This transition from recruited average unfit citizen to the physically fit Royal Marines Commando is a tribute to the potential and resilience of the human body. The secret is physical exercise.

The lesson is that given motivation and the opportunity, the body can realise a degree of its physical potential. The better the physical make-up of any body, the greater the potential. Coaching and practice will give the necessary techniques that turn the potential into achievement on the track, water or field.

One of the key words to this healthy mixture is "motivation", for without the motivation of "will" to accept the challenge, the challenge cannot exist. We offer a challenge to those whose fitness level is much higher than an average member of the public and to those of this group who feel that they need something more taxing and energetic than the level of physical fitness we have hitherto suggested.

It is difficult to be specific about any level of fitness higher than normal fitness (super fitness) and even more it is difficult to design an accurate test, because there are several types of fitness. These are listed as follows:

(a) Muscular endurance: the ability of a group of muscles to delay the onset of fatigue.
(b) Local muscular endurance: the ability of a single muscle to delay the onset of fatigue.
(c) Total endurance: the ability of the body as a whole to delay the onset of fatigue.
(d) Cardio-respiratory fitness: the ability of the heart and lungs to work efficiently together for as long as possible under physical stress.

From these definitions it is easy to adduce that the heavyweight weight-lifter will have a different bias to the fitness from that for which a long-distance runner aims. The weight-lifter will have trained his muscles to respond to short explosive bursts, whereas the cross-country runner will have trained to endure hard work for long spells.

It is because of the variation in types of fitness that we only offer some possible ideas.

The first is an old test which has been used in the Services to give a general guide to fitness. The test is:

1. Pull ups   Maximum 18
2. Press ups   Maximum 60
3. Sit ups   Maximum 85 in 2 minutes
4. Burpees   Maximum 41 in one minute
5. Shuttle run   5 × 60 yards in under 44 seconds.

This test should be done in the listed order, with only a two-minute rest between each activity. You can always try this test if you are very fit and give yourself the challenge of improving your score. If you can reach the maximum in all five tests, without cheating, then you can reckon yourself to be in the super-fit class.

One of the tests which was given to a Royal Marines Physical Training Instructors Class at the end of a course of sixteen weeks is given below, with the instructor's comments:

1. Pull ups   14 is very good—"The best I've seen is 52". World record 78.
2. Press ups   40 is very good—"The best I've seen is 129".
3. Sit ups   60 is very good—"The best I've seen is 580".
   (no pause)
4. Burpees   35 is very good in a minute—"The best I've seen is 44".

There are many other physical tests which are incredibly hard to do and which certainly present a challenge. We list three such tests for interest:

1. Hand stand press ups—one is very good, "I have seen 17".
2. Dips in parallel bars—30 is very good, "I have seen 101".
3. High V sits—40 is very good, "I have seen 75".

The majority of the exercises listed so far are muscular endurance type tests. They should only be tried by the fanatic and anybody who gets into the very good class is achieving a remarkable standard. The fact that you cannot attempt such things as "hand stand press ups" does not mean that you are not physically fit. One of the authors is physically fit, but can barely do a handstand, let alone do press ups from that position!

Fitness in specific sports is relevant to overall fitness, but it is difficult to give a test which will prove a suitable challenge to the gladiator, because the requirements, skills and indeed demands on the body vary from sport to sport. It is probably more useful for the sportsman to design his own test, basing it on the relevant physical demands to a particular sport. We content ourselves by suggesting a good example of a test sometimes used to assess fitness in team games such as basketball, football, hockey and rugby football. It is:

(a) Mark out 25 yards in sections of five yards.
(b) Run to the five-yard mark and return to the start, then run to the ten-yard mark and back, then to the fifteen, then to the twenty and finally to the twenty-five mark and back to the start line.
(c) Take your running time for the "circuit", stop the watch for thirty-five seconds while you rest and your pulse starts its recovery period.
(d) Do five more of these circuits, making six runs and five rest periods.
(e) Take the overall running time, which should be somewhere around the 200-second mark.

(f) A scale score is: 216 Fair
210 Adequate
204 Good
198 Very good
192 Excellent
188 Superb
184 Supreme
180 Incredible!

This is a tortuous test which is both hard work and pretty accurate. The easiest way to set this up is to mark the yards on string which you can then lay whenever you want either a test or some remarkably effective exercise.

Another test which will provide a challenge to the really super fit is simply four basic tests. Each one will present the male with a challenge on its own, but combined, and if done in half an hour, will present a major challenge. The tests are:

1. Sit ups: over 60 in two minutes.
2. Press ups: over 50 without pause.
3. Burpees: over 35 in a minute.
4. One mile run in under 5 minutes 30 seconds.

Amongst the suggested tests listed in this chapter are the sort of levels to which the ordinary young human male might aim if he was particularly interested in some sort of strength and endurance target. For the active sportsman the challenge can more usefully be set by the coach or instructor and it is evident that some of the tests we have listed are both beyond and even irrelevant to the average week-end sportsman.

In discussing the super fit we have deliberately left out any reference to physical challenges for women, because we feel that the sort of woman interested in fitness targets is probably a participant sportswoman. In this event, we suggest that she should consult her coach and get her challenge from the stopwatch, the tape measure or the record book.

It must be understood that the challenges of the type we have outlined are not necessary to this book, but rather add a little spice to the fare offered to the real enthusiast. It also serves to show something of the realm that lies beyond normal fitness. It is enough just to be physically fit.

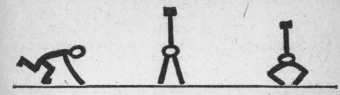

Hand-stand press ups

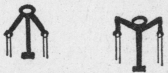

Dips

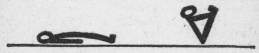

High V sits

Pull ups

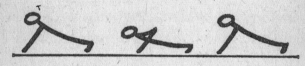

Press ups

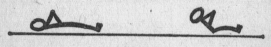

Sit ups

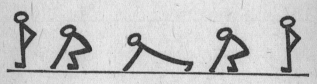

Burpees

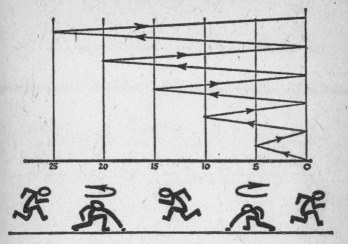

Shuttle runs

CHAPTER X

POSTSCRIPT TO A FITNESS PLAN

This book has had a simple aim. This aim has been to make you aware of the importance of being physically fit, to provide you with the basic knowledge of what being physically fit means and to present you with a plan which you can use to become and to keep fit.

Although much has been said and written on the subject before, we believe that the time is right for the practical physical trainer, rather than the highly qualified theorist, to interpret the mountain of knowledge which overshadows and appears not to influence a dangerously under-exercised society. We offer our practical knowledge and present our ideas, in the hope that many of you will understand something which is vital to your health today and life ahead.

"Fitness breeds confidence" is to be found in many a sportsman's vocabulary and we are confident that our message will be recognised as important. We believe that this book offers a chance to many, who might otherwise not be aware of how to see and seek a healthier and happier life.

PEAR'S MEDICAL ENCYCLOPAEDIA

J. A. C. BROWN MB, BChir.

The aim of PEAR'S MEDICAL ENCYCLOPAEDIA is to
encourage co-operation between doctor and patient by
presenting sensible articles on medical matters and providing
an essential reference book for good health in the home.
Obviously the book cannot take the place of a doctor's
professional care, but it *can* provide the layman (and the
nurse or student doctor) with reasonably detailed scientific
information and helpful advice. As a popular guide, in
sickness and in health, it has been an invaluable standby in
hundreds of thousands of homes for many years. The revised
edition, besides dealing sympathetically with the perennial
worrying questions, includes entries concerning
contemporary topics such as the Pill, heart transplants,
the kidney machine and mouth-to-mouth resuscitation. In
this new edition PEAR'S MEDICAL ENCYCLOPAEDIA
also becomes truly international, covering tropical diseases
and providing advice for travellers.

Health And Medicine   0 7221 1908 9   £2.95

A GUIDE TO SQUASH

RICHARD HAWKEY

Squash has always been popular, but recently it has enjoyed a tremendous boom throughout the world. This upsurge of interest is understandable, for squash fits so well into our modern lifestyle. It is such a concentrated form of exercise that it does not demand all one's spare time to stay fit; the game is played indoors, so one is not dependent on good weather or natural light; and the equipment is simple and inexpensive – a racket and one ball.

A GUIDE TO SQUASH presents all the necessary tactics, strokes and rules of the game for match play. In addition there is a brief history of squash, together with hints on training and fitness. The instruction given follows that approved for the Squash Rackets Association's amateur coaches – who are taught and examined for their qualifications by Richard Hawkey, the author of the book.

Fully Illustrated

Sports And Hobbies   0 7221 4415 6   85p

EASY YOGA EXERCISES

WILLIAM ZORN

William Zorn has presented systematically and explained clearly the simpler techniques of yoga, especially for beginners, in EASY YOGA EXERCISES – a book aimed at all age groups. Yoga can be tremendously benefiting, and he shows you how to do it without tying yourself in knots or viewing the world from an upside down position.

Eating habits have a large part to play in the fitness and health of your body and you can learn about proteins, vitamins and minerals, and know the foods in which these all-important substances are found. There is also a chapter on slimming the sensible and lasting way.

Yoga   *Illustrated*   0 7221 9437 4   75p

A MAN CALLED INTREPID:
The Secret War 1939–1945

WILLIAM STEVENSON

A MAN CALLED INTREPID tells for the first time the full story of British Security Co-ordination, the international Allied intelligence agency of World War Two whose work has been a closely guarded secret for the past thirty years. Here are top-level inside accounts of crucial wartime undercover operations including:

The breaking of the German *Enigma* code
The assassination of Heydrich
The race for the atomic bomb
Surveillance and sabotage of Nazi V1 and V2 rocket sites
The raids on the French coast that made the Normandy landings possible
Anglo-American co-operation in the sinking of the *Bismarck*
The organization of resistance movements throughout Europe
The intelligence stratagems that delayed the Nazi invasion of Russia

Written with full access to all the British Security Co-ordination papers and with the full co-operation of BSC's director, the man code-named INTREPID, William Stevenson's internationally bestselling book is a uniquely important piece of modern secret history. It is also tremendously exciting to read.

'A work of profound historical importance ... a great adventure story, wherein fact is more sensational than fiction .. more stimulating than any record I have seen about the infinite complexity of modern warfare'

> David Bruce
> (Former OSS chief and later US Ambassador to Britain)

Biography/War   07221 8159 0   £1.75

A selection of Bestsellers from Sphere Books

Fiction

THE DEATH FREAK	John Luckless	95p
BEL RIA	Sheila Burnford	95p
WOLFSBANE	Craig Thomas	£1.25p
GOODBYE	W. H. Manville	£1.25p
GOLDEN MOMENTS	Danielle Steel	£1.25p

Film and TV Tie-ins

THE PROFESSIONALS 5: BLIND RUN	Ken Blake	85p
THE PROFESSIONALS 6: FALL GIRL	Ken Blake	85p
THE MUSIC MACHINE	Bill Stoddart	95p
THE PROMISE	Danielle Steel	95p
BUCK ROGERS IN THE 25th CENTURY	Addison E. Steele	95p
BUCK ROGERS 2: THAT MAN ON BETA	Addison E. Steele	95p

Non-Fiction

THE THIRD WORLD WAR	General Sir John Hackett	£1.75p
INSIDE THE FOURTH REICH	Eric Erdstein	95p
THE CONVICT	Felix Milani	£1.25p
COME WIND OR WEATHER	Clare Francis	95p

All Sphere books are available at your local bookshop or newsagent, c can be ordered direct from the publisher. Just tick the titles you wan and fill in the form below.

Name...

Address..

....

Write to Sphere Books, Cash Sales Department, P.O. Box 11, Falmout! Cornwall TR10 9EN

Please enclose cheque or postal order to the value of the cover price plu

UK: 25p for the first book plus 10p per copy for each additional boc ordered to a maximum charge of £1.05.

OVERSEAS: 40p for the first book and 12p for each additional book.

BFPO & EIRE: 25p for the first book plus 10p per copy for the ne 8 books, thereafter 5p per book.

Sphere Books reserve the right to show new retail prices on covers whi may differ from those previously advertised in the text or elsewhere, a to increase postal rates in accordance with the GPO.

(8: